THE
COMMON
C0LD
CURE

Ray Sahelian, MD
Victoria Dolby Toews, MPH

AVERY PUBLISHING GROUP

Garden City Park • New York

The therapeutic procedures presented in this book are based on the research, training, and personal experience of the authors, and are true and complete to the best of the authors' knowledge. This book is intended as an informative guide. It is not intended to replace or countermand the advice given to you by your physician. Because each person and each situation is unique, the publisher urges the reader to check with a qualified health professional before using any procedure or remedy where there is any question regarding appropriateness.

The publisher does not advocate the use of any particular herbal remedy, supplement program, or dietary regimen, but believes that the information presented in this book should be available to the public. Because there is always some risk involved, the authors and publisher are not responsible for any adverse effects or consequences resulting from the use of any of the suggestions in this book. Please feel free to consult a physician or other qualified health professional. It is a sign of wisdom, not cowardice, to seek a second or third opinion.

Cover designer: Eric Macaluso
Editor: Helene Ciaravino
Typesetter: Gary A. Rosenberg
Printer: Paragon Press, Honesdale, PA

Avery Publishing Group
120 Old Broadway
Garden City Park, NY 11040
1–800–548–5757
www.averypublishing.com

Library of Congress Cataloging-in-Publication Data

Sahelian, Ray.
        The common cold cure: natural remedies for colds and flu /
    by Ray Sahelian and Victoria Dolby Toews.
            p.   cm.
        Includes bibliographical references and index.
        ISBN 0–89529–882–1
        1. Cold (Disease)—Popular works.   2. Influenza—Popular works.
3. Cold (Disease)—Alternative treatment. 4. Influenza—Alternative
    treatment. 5. Naturopathy.   I. Dolby Toews, Victoria.   II. Title.
    RF361.S24 1999
    616.2'05—dc21   98-32415
                                                          CIP

Printed in the United States of America.

10 9 8 7 6 5 4 3 2 1

Contents

To my mom —

Thanks for the TLC through my childhood colds, and ever since.

You're the best!

— VDT

Introduction

*T*he *Common Cold Cure.* Upon first hearing this title, you may think it sounds like a promise we can't live up to. But considering the fact that both authors of this book and many of Dr. Sahelian's patients have not experienced a full-blown cold or flu in many years—simply by applying the natural ways to prevent and fight infections shared in this book—this title might not be so farfetched afterall.

Short of hibernating in your house all winter and avoiding human contact, there is no way to avoid exposure to the viruses that cause the oh-so-common cold and influenza. As hard as you try to evade these viruses, they're lying in wait everywhere you go and on everything you touch—the hand you shook, the doorknob you turned, the keypad at the bank machine. In short, there's probably a cold or flu virus with your name on it somewhere this winter season. But you—like us—can enjoy good health during the cold and flu season by following the advice in the chapters to come.

We'll start out by explaining, in Chapter 1, how your immune system works, specific details about cold and flu viruses, and the dietary and lifestyle factors that can work either for or against optimal immunity. In Chapter 2, we'll delve into the conventional treatments for colds and flu. In Chapters 3, 4, and 5, the attention turns to vitamin C, zinc, and echinacea, respectively—the top three natural cold fighters. Chapter 6 thoroughly reviews many other herbs that have both traditional and/or scientific evidence for supporting the immune system and fighting infection.

If you currently have a cold or flu, you might want to flip right to Chapter 7, where you'll find in-depth guidelines for going on the nutritional defensive. Actually, the information is important for both the treatment and prevention of colds and the flu. You'll find concrete tips about how to maximize your immune function to fend off germs. And in case a germ makes it through your immune defenses, there's plenty of advice to get you on the nutritional offensive so that you can halt an infection in its tracks. Furthermore, Chapter 7 includes special sections geared to the needs of kids and travelers—two groups who suffer through more than their fair share of colds and flus. Finally, Chapter 8 gives a breakdown, symptom by symptom, of many natural ways to lessen your discomfort when you're in the throes of an upper respiratory infection.

The strategies shared in this book really do work. Take note of this real-world example that one of us experienced during a recent winter:

Dr. Sahelian awoke one winter morning at 5 A.M. with a slightly congested nose and a fullness in the throat. Two days earlier, one of the employees at his office had come in with symptoms of a cold, including a runny nose, sneezing, and coughing. Thinking that perhaps that was the source of his exposure to a cold virus, Dr. Sahelian wanted to take full preventive action before it progressed any further.

Dr. Sahelian immediately went to the kitchen (where he keeps all of his supplements) and swallowed ten vitamin C pills, each containing 500 milligrams. He put the tea kettle on and, while the water was heating, dropped a zinc lozenge in his mouth. As soon as it melted, Dr. Sahelian took another lozenge. By now the water was boiling. The doctor placed two tea bags of echinacea in a large glass, added a couple of drops of stevia sweetener, and poured in the boiling water. He finished the tea over the next ten minutes and then popped a third zinc lozenge into his mouth. Within two hours, the slight congestion in Dr. Sahelian's nose and the fullness in his throat had disappeared. He believes the unlucky virus that had attempted to settle in the mucous membranes of his nose and throat had been promptly zapped to annihilation. To attain the same success in fighting colds and flu as Dr. Sahelian, follow the step-by-step guide on pages 107 to 114.

Such is the power of the natural supplements you'll find described throughout this book. We aim at providing you with safe, effective, natural ways to get through the cold and flu season without the usual coughs and congestion. If you follow the advice that we present in this and the following chapters, your risk of catching a cold or the flu will be dramatically reduced. And even if you do catch a bug, you will be able to minimize the annoying symptoms. You and your family can make it through future cold and flu seasons happier and healthier. So turn the page and start learning how to bolster your defenses. Make this a year of victory over the viruses that cause the common cold and flu!

1

Boost Your Immune System and Beat the Bugs

They're everywhere—on your skin, in the tub, on the kitchen sink. They're lurking between the fingers of the person you shook hands with, floating in the air, and even lounging in the fruit salad. And they're looking for you, tracking and hunting you down in order to make you their next victim. You can't hide from them.

No, you're not paranoid. This is the reality. Disease bugs are everywhere, even thriving several feet under the Antarctic ice and within boiling natural springs. But don't be too terrified. Over millions of years of evolution, the human body has developed a good relationship with many of the bugs on this planet. Hundreds of different bacteria now live in harmony with your body, as permanent residents in your gut, helping to break down some foodstuffs and even helping to make nutrients such as the vitamin biotin. And any bugs that are your enemies have quite a challenge to overcome: the highly evolved and powerful human immune system.

Even considering the wonderful way in which the immune system fights off invaders, some bugs will find ways to penetrate the defenses. A major premise of *The Common Cold Cure* rests on ways to boost the power of the immune system in order not to give these bugs the opportunity to make an effective landing on your respiratory tissues. If they do land and try to get a foothold, your strengthened immune system can swiftly give them the boot. And if by great persistence they do start making inroads, many of the nutrients discussed in this book will batter them unconscious. Let's start with learning some basic facts about our natural defenses and how we can help them to function better.

THE IMMUNE SYSTEM

Dr. Sahelian went through the normal process of medical education and residency just as all medical students do. He was taught about the immune system—how T cells work, the role of the spleen and the thymus gland, and many of the intricate details of this complicated system. But he doesn't recall ever being taught how to *improve* the immune system. It was always assumed that if you left it alone, the immune system would function optimally. There was no reason to think that any nutritional manipulation could influence it. In fact, Dr. Sahelian remembers asking his immunology professor if there were any dietary or nutritional changes we could make to boost the fighting power of immune cells. The professor's blank stare showed that this was the first time he had ever even entertained the thought.

As Dr. Sahelian continued his medical education, he fell into the traditional medical trap of thinking that a specific antibiotic, antiviral, or antiparasitic medicine was the only option in treating infectious diseases. Although such medicines have enormous benefits in treating and curing many of the infections that previously incapacitated or killed countless people, they are not the only answer. Many of the individuals who are afflicted with infectious agents have weak immune systems. Instead of focusing exclusively on killing the germ, why not take a more comprehensive approach by finding ways to stimulate the immune system to do some of its own killing of these undesirable intruders?

Although traditional medicine has advanced by leaps and bounds in certain areas, it is still in the Middle Ages when it comes to incorporating nutritional and immune-boosting approaches to its armaments. But we're living in an exciting age—a revolution has started with consumers demanding that their physicians learn about and keep up with natural approaches and alternatives to toxic drugs. We're finding natural, healthy ways to make our bodies better fighters. The immune system *can* be improved.

The Birth of the Immune System

The primary purpose of the immune system is to prevent unfriendly germs from getting a foothold in the body. The maturing process of the immune system begins in the womb. Within the bone marrow of the fetus, a single primitive type of cell called the *stem cell* begins to differentiate into *lymphoid cells* and *myeloid cells*, which go on to form additional cells of the immune system.

Lymphoid stem cells mature into T lymphocytes, B lymphocytes, and natural killer cells. All of these are white blood cells. T lymphocytes are so called because they first go to the thymus gland (hence the "T") in order to mature. B lymphocytes are so called because they remain in the bone marrow (hence the "B") in order to continue with their development. Finally, the natural killer cells are lymphocytes that serve in the active fight against viruses and cancer cells.

Myeloid stem cells mature into neutrophils, eosinophils, and red blood cells. Neutrophils are the most abundant type of white blood cells, which fight disease and infection. Eosinophils are responsible for killing parasites and are also involved in allergic reactions. Finally, red blood cells carry the oxygen that is needed to feed our tissues and organs. (See Figure 1.1.)

The Immune System After Birth

At about the time of birth, the immune system has almost fully matured. A number of immune cells are now present in the blood, thymus gland, spleen, skin, mucous membranes, and the lymphatic system. It is absolutely necessary that the immune system be developed by birth, for otherwise the vulnerable infant would quickly fall prey to the countless germs of our environment. Breastfeeding is extremely important, since breastmilk contains a number of immune components, such as immunoglobulins, that are not present in formula. These components bolster the infant's resistance to infection.

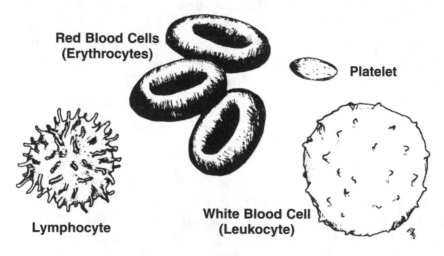

Red Blood Cells
(Erythrocytes)

Platelet

Lymphocyte

White Blood Cell
(Leukocyte)

Figure 1.1. Cells Found in the Blood

During the first few months and years of life, infants and children are constantly exposed to new viruses and bacteria. Each germ has specific proteins or compounds, called *antigens*, that can be recognized by the immune system. With each exposure, the T and B lymphocytes mount an attack by making and releasing *antibodies*, which are proteins that attach to the antigens, making it easier to destroy the foreign substance. Once the immune system makes antibodies against these antigens, it remembers (almost forever) how to make them again very quickly when re-exposed to the germ. Hence, as we get older, we tend to come down with fewer colds and infections because the immune system can quickly put out specific antibodies that thwart the invading germ.

THE COMMON COLD

As you may already know, the word *rhino* means "nose." It follows that *rhinoviruses* are viruses that infect the upper respiratory system, which includes the nose, sinuses, mouth, and throat (pharynx). Upper respiratory infections, referred to as URIs, are the most common acute illnesses in the United States and the Western world. They constitute what are referred to as common colds. The usual symptoms of the common cold are nasal discharge and obstruction, sneezing, sore throat, cough, and hoarseness.

Although URIs can be caused by bacteria, viruses are much more likely culprits. There are at least 200 different viruses that cause colds. Most of these are rhinoviruses, but coronaviruses, influenza, and other types also cause URIs.

The Symptoms

Once the cold virus gets a foothold in the upper respiratory system, a person begins to experience symptoms within two to three days. The earliest symptoms are a feeling of uneasiness or malaise, sneezing, runny nose, scratchy throat, slight fever, and a decrease in the senses of smell and taste. These symptoms get worse over the next two to four days, and it is during this time that transmission of the virus to another person is most likely. Later symptoms of a cold include hoarseness and cough. Most symptoms last one week, but in certain individuals they can go on for two weeks. Sometimes a dry cough is the last symptom to go away.

For practical purposes, it is not necessary to identify the exact type of virus causing a particular cold. The most important role for a physician is to make sure the cold has not progressed to a more severe infection. Sometimes the damage to the upper respiratory lining from the cold virus allows more virulent germs to attack, and then a simple cold can turn into a bacterial infection. Such an infection can spread to the sinuses and lead to sinusitis, go through the Eustachian tubes to cause an ear infection, or progress down to the lower respiratory tract and result in pneumonia. (The lower respiratory system includes the trachea and the lungs.) A secondary infection by a more virulent bug is more likely to occur in certain populations: children; the elderly; individuals who have existing lung diseases, such as those with asthma or emphysema; individuals who have compromised immune systems, such as those with AIDS; and individuals who are on medicines that interfere with immunity, such as prednisone.

Resistance Over Time

When Dr. Sahelian started his medical internship back in 1984, he often came down with colds—particularly when he worked in the pediatric unit. Internship was a stressful time and the doctor always seemed to be sleep deprived. And on top of everything else, the hospital food wasn't that healthy. Hence, the combination of a poor diet, lack of sleep, stress, and exposure to children with infections was enough to overwhelm his immune system. Yet as the residency progressed, even though the stress continued, Dr. Sahelian didn't seem to come down with colds as frequently. Apparently he had become exposed to quite a number of bugs and had built up antibodies against them. Usually, doctors who have been in practice for many years rarely come down with colds because they have been exposed to almost all of the different types of rhinoviruses.

Most adults come down with a cold between two and four times a year, while children usually average six to eight colds a year. Since the most common way to transmit a cold is through human contact, most families are exposed to cold viruses through children who bring them home from school. Daycare centers, in particular, are hotbeds for colds. The children are in close proximity, and they often touch each other on the hands and face before and after rubbing their own noses. Cold viruses can survive on the body or hands for several hours, during which time contact with another person gives the virus a free ride. Although viruses can be transmitted through the air, hand-to-hand contact is the most reliable way to transmit these bugs. Many of Dr. Sahelian's adult patients report that the incidence of colds in the family rose dramatically after their children were placed in daycare centers.

Over time, most individuals are exposed to a number of common cold viruses and do not easily succumb to them during subsequent exposure. The odds of catching a cold are thus reduced with age, except for the senior population, as their immune systems often begin to falter.

THE DREADED FLU

The most common cause of the flu is the influenza virus, although other viruses, such as parainfluenza and adenovirus, produce similar symptoms. The two most common types of the influenza virus are identified as types A and B and are clinically indistinguishable. Although there are exceptions, most cases usually occur in an epidemic pattern at varying intervals, usually in the fall and winter. It is difficult to diagnose influenza in the absence of an epidemic, since the disease resembles many other mild, fever-producing illnesses.

The Symptoms

Although there's a good amount of overlap in symptoms between the common cold and the flu, these two types of illness differ in some major aspects. The flu syndrome comes on abruptly and causes weakness, tiredness, muscle aches, headache, and fever. Unlike the common cold, during which a person's temperature elevates by only about one degree, the flu virus can cause temperature elevations of up to five or six degrees. Furthermore, the flu is almost always accompanied by a cough. Muscle aches can occur in the lower back, thighs, and arms. There can even be pain behind the eyes.

The flu viruses cause much more misery than the common cold viruses. A person who is suffering from a flu feels like all of the energy has been drained out of him or her. Some individuals even suffer from temporary depression. One of the last symptoms to go away is a cough that can persist for weeks afterwards.

Unlike the common cold, which is transmitted mostly through hand-to-hand contact, the most common way influenza is transmitted is through small particle aerosols in the air that are dispersed by sneezing, coughing, and talking. Once the flu virus gets a foothold, symptoms can start as soon as twelve hours and as late as three days after exposure. Transmission of the virus to another person most often occurs during the first three days after the onset of the flu symptoms.

Flu Vaccinations

Each year, flu viruses can undergo slight variations in their protein structures, thus making the antibodies that the body made in the previous year practically ineffective. So at the beginning of each flu season, a committee at the Food and Drug Administration (FDA) determines the types of changes the flu viruses have undergone and recommends a new vaccine. The vaccines help individuals who are at risk for the flu to mount a more effective defense.

Flu vaccines are often given in October and November. They can protect certain individuals with weak immune systems. Good candidates for flu vaccinations are the elderly, those with chronic heart or lung conditions, and certain health-care workers. However, there are also reasons why a vaccine is less than ideal when it comes to fighting off the flu. See pages 26 to 27 for more information.

THE TOP FOUR IMMUNE BUSTERS

Why are some people seemingly immune to colds and the flu, while others have to carry around the tissue box as if it were a teddy bear? Quite a number of factors influence the immune system. Of course, we cannot discount genetics. Some people are lucky to be born with highly evolved immune systems. And then we must take into consideration each child's nutritional development during the stages when the immune system is completing development. Usually, the healthiest babies are those whose mothers had excellent nutritional habits and breastfed them as infants, and whose parents cooked great meals with plenty of wholesome foods and fresh produce.

Notwithstanding genetics and early childhood diet, quite a number of factors can influence a person's current immune status. Over the years, we have observed four common factors that increase a person's risk of coming down with colds and the flu: lack of adequate sleep; stress; poor diet; and smoking.

Lack of Adequate Sleep

We cannot emphasize enough the importance of good, regular, deep sleep. It plays an integral role in proper immune system function. Many of the immune cells, such as natural killer cells, are activated during deep sleep. The first question Dr. Sahelian asks a patient who comes into the office with cold symptoms is, "How are you sleeping at night?" In most cases, the patient will report some event that disrupted his or her sleep patterns, whether it be traveling through different time zones on a recent trip, changing a work schedule, or staying up late at parties. The body cannot recuperate without adequate rest.

Stress

Another common cause of immune dysfunction is stress, whether it be psychological (such as relationship difficulties and financial worries) or physical (for example, intense athletic competition and illness). Stress definitely has harmful biological effects. The immune system responds quickly to thoughts and emotions. There are receptors on the surface of white blood cells to which hormones and neurotransmitters attach. When under stress, substances released by the brain attach to these receptors and disturb the cells' regular functioning. The immune system can, in turn, send substances back to the brain, altering the release of neurotransmitters and influencing mood and cognition. At the other end of the spectrum, positive thoughts and emotions are, in some instances, believed to enhance the immune system.

Luckily, we can do something about stress. Much of it is self-induced or self-aggravated. While stuck in traffic, we can either boil with frustration or turn on the radio and hum along with the songs. Most of our daily stress is not necessarily due to external circumstances. Rather it is due to our underdeveloped coping skills.

Poor Diet

Walk into any grocery store and you'll see stacks of sodas, potato chips, cookies, and pies within impulse reach. Countless Americans thoughtlessly place these convenience junk foods in their shopping carts at the expense of nutritious foods. There is no doubt that the immune system cannot function at its best when constantly exposed to this junk. Such food is often devoid of vitamins, minerals, and nutrients necessary for the proper function of the immune system. Furthermore, the high levels of sugar and processed fats in junk food interfere with immunity. Having said that, if you normally have a good diet, don't feel guilty for occasionally eating desserts or munching on a convenience food. See this chapter's section on "Healthy Eating Habits" for some good dietary advice.

Smoking

Cigarette smoking can damage the lining of the respiratory system. When that lining is impaired, the risk increases for germs to gain a foothold. Cigarette smoke contains many toxic chemicals that damage the *cilia*—hairlike structures that line the respiratory system and constantly sweep out germs that have been inhaled. As a result, smoking could well increase your risk of catching a cold.

HEALTHY EATING HABITS

Much has been written about healthy eating habits. The basics include several easy-to-follow guidelines. First, reduce your intake of sugar and simple carbohydrates. Use the natural, no-calorie sweetener *stevia* as a partial substitute for sugar. Also, decrease your intake of fried foods, margarine, and baked goods. These foods contain trans-fatty acids and hydrogenated oils that interfere with the function of good fats. Fats make up the lining of white blood cells. If this lining includes healthy fats from whole foods and fish, the immune cells are able to function better.

Be sure to include more omega-3 fatty acids in the diet, particularly through consumption of cold-water fish. If you don't eat much fish and other marine products, take supplements of DHA and EPA, which are two forms of omega-3s. In addition, use more olive, canola, and flaxseed oils, and less safflower, sunflower, and corn oils, in order to get the right type of fatty acids. These fatty acids can improve the function of immune cells by making the cell membranes more fluid and by enabling the immune cells to detect germs more easily.

Vary your fruit and vegetable intakes by purchasing produce that you don't normally eat. Each fruit or vegetable has a unique set of carotenoids and flavonoids. These plant chemicals have powerful antiviral and antibacterial effects. They also have anti-inflammatory abilities that can reduce the risk for allergies. And be sure to add garlic or onions to your salads or other dishes, since they have antiviral components.

It is very important to drink plenty of fluids throughout the day. This will keep your system cleansed and well-hydrated. Drink one or two large glasses of water when you wake up in the morning, to help empty the colon. Furthermore, drink a variety of herbal teas instead of just regular tea or coffee. Each morning, have a different type of tea, such as ginger, green tea, licorice, peppermint, or elderberry. Herbs contain a number of compounds that fight germs. For more information, see Chapter 6.

Finally, at least two or three times a week, add yogurt with active cultures to your diet. The bacteria in yogurt colonize the gut to prevent harmful germs from getting a foothold. These tips should get you started on your way to a stronger immune system. Dietary changes can make a large difference in your body's ability to beat the bugs.

IMPORTANT IMMUNE-BOOSTING SUPPLEMENTS

In addition to direct dietary changes, you can enhance your nutrition with supplements. Before you begin supplementation, make sure you first have good lifestyle habits, including proper sleep, good diet, exercise, and stress-reduction techniques. Once you have your basic foundation, you can explore the benefits of natural supplements as adjuncts to immune stimulation. We recommend the following nutrients, especially during the winter season:

- Vitamin C, 100 to 250 milligrams once or twice a day.

- A multivitamin supplement supplying one to two times the RDA for the B vitamins.

- Vitamin E, 30 to 200 international units (IU) per day.

- A multimineral supplement supplying 50 to 100 percent of the RDA for minerals.

- Fish oil capsules supplying between 500 and 1,000 milligrams of DHA and EPA, if you don't normally eat fish. If you are a strict vegetarian and do not want to take fish oil capsules, take a teaspoonful of flax oil daily.

- Probiotics, if you're not a yogurt eater. These probiotics contain beneficial bacteria, such as acidophilus and bifidobacteria. (If you do include yogurt in your diet, this supplement is not necessary.)

- Garlic pills, one or two capsules a day, if you don't normally consume garlic.

- Melatonin, 0.3 to 0.5 milligrams once or twice a week, an hour or two before bed. This substance is helpful if you have trouble sleeping. Remember, deep sleep rejuvenates the immune system.

CONCLUSION

There is no doubt that if you adopt the healthy lifestyle habits of proper sleep, adequate exercise, nourishing foods, and stress management, your risk for catching the cold or flu will decrease dramatically. Taking additional supplements can provide you with extra protection. Suffering from a few bouts of the common cold or the flu each season is not inevitable. Beat the viruses from the very beginning by boosting your immune system. It's much more preferable than attempting to smother the symptoms once your body has been invaded.

2 Conventional Medicine Versus the Common Cold and Flu

C onventional medicine offers several approaches for cold care, but its quick fixes are often not the best avenue to take. This chapter discusses the ups and downs of the substances typically used in orthodox methods of treating the common cold and the flu. In general, conventional medicine's approach is that there is no real remedy for the common cold and flu, that there are only agents of symptom relief.

During a visit at his parents' house for dinner, Dr. Sahelian mentioned that he was writing a book about colds and flu. Harry, the doctor's dad, likes to tell jokes. He told this one about doctors and treating colds:

A patient went to his doctor because he was suffering from a cold. The doctor said, "Sorry, but I don't have a cure for the common cold."

"What do you advise then, Doc?" the patient asked.

"I recommend that you take a long, hot bath," said the doctor.

"That's a good idea. Then what?"

"After you come out of the hot bath, don't dry yourself. Just walk over to the living room window, open it completely, allow the frigid air to blow in, stretch your arms and legs, and take deep breaths in and out until you start shivering."

"What! That could well enough turn my cold into a pneumonia!" exclaimed the patient.

"That's the idea!" said the doctor, "Now, pneumonia I have a cure for."

PRESCRIPTIONS THAT APPEASE THE PATIENT

Doctors have a difficult dilemma when it comes to treating the common cold. Typically, when a person catches a cold, he or she first tries nonprescription pharmaceutical agents for a couple of days before giving up and scheduling an office visit with a doctor. By this time, the cold virus has comfortably settled in and is not willing to budge for another week, no matter what. Most doctors who practice conventional medicine will inform their patients that there are no great ways to treat the common cold. They typically recommend some over-the-counter decongestants or antihistamines for symptom relief. However, patients are rarely happy with this advice. They don't make the effort to come all the way to the office and to pay a considerable sum just to be told to take over-the-counter pills. Sensing this frustration, many doctors will reluctantly pull out a pad and write down a prescription for an antibiotic.

Another reason doctors quickly prescribe antibiotics is because of our current medico-legal system. Doctors are afraid that if they miss underlying bacterial infections that are brewing, they'll get nasty letters from the patients' lawyers. The threat of litigation now hangs over every medical visit. So some physicians feel that prescribing possibly unnecessary antibiotics is the safer bet, when compared with overlooking a potentially serious infection. It is important to state that physicians do sometimes justifiably prescribe the antibiotics, if they are concerned that the patient already has a condition—such as asthma or a compromised immune system—that could be aggravated if a bacterial infection joins the viral infection.

Studies have shown that even though viruses cause 90 percent of upper respiratory infections, at least half of all patients with colds receive prescriptions for antibiotics. Many patients don't realize that antibiotics don't kill viruses, and they are satisfied since they now have a prescription. I've been guilty of writing prescriptions to appease patients in the past. Chances are the cold symptoms will last just as many days with the antibiotic treatment as they will without the antibiotics. But, by giving the prescription, the doctor saves himself or herself a phone call, over the next day or two, from an angry patient whose symptoms have not improved. The patient is often upset at not having received a prescription medication after paying for an office visit.

Unfortunately, this misprescribing is a leading cause of the emerging problem of antibiotic resistance in the United States. In the 1970s, close to 100 percent of throat infections caused by the streptococcus bacteria were susceptible to penicillin. Now, 40 percent or more of these bacteria are resistant to penicillin. The indiscriminate use of antibiotics can also lead to common side effects. These include diarrhea, yeast infections, fatigue, and allergic reactions. So don't bother taking antibiotics for viral infections or allergies, as they do not help and may even do harm.

THE CONFUSING "COLD RELIEF" AISLE AT THE DRUGSTORE

Your nose is congested, your throat hurts, and you feel a slight fever coming on. You drop by your local drug store to get some relief before things take a turn for the worse. If you thought choosing the best shampoo was difficult from all of the options available on the shelves, just try to make the right choice from the hundreds of different cold and flu products! In order to simplify matters, we can categorize cold medicines into seven categories: antifever medicines;

Is It a Virus, Bacteria, or an Allergy?

*When common upper respiratory symptoms occur—runny nose, sore throat, congestion, etc.—it can be difficult to identify the source. Did you catch a virus? Did bacteria invade you? Are you allergic to something in the air? The following explanations will help you figure out what kind of irritant is behind your misery. By knowing the type of attack, you can better manage your illness. Keep in mind that viral infections and allergies **do not** improve with antibiotic treatments.*

Symptom	Virus	Bacteria	Allergy
Fever	Common	Common	Never
Runny nose	Common	Rare	Common
Nasal congestion	Common	Rare	Common
Muscle aches/pains	Common	Rare	Never
Headache	Common	Sometimes	Never
Cough	Common	Sometimes	Rare
Dry cough	Common	Rare	Sometimes
Clear mucus	Common	Rare	Sometimes
Yellow/Green mucus	Sometimes	Common	Never
Hoarse voice	Common	Rare	Sometimes
Seasonal symptoms	Sometimes	Rare	Common

decongestants; antihistamines; pain medicines (analgesics); cough suppressants; expectorants; and sore-throat relief medicines. Keep in mind that, unlike natural supplements, none of these medicines reduce the length of a cold. Also, it is important to remember that individuals who are pregnant should consult a doctor before taking any medication.

Antifever Medicines

Aspirin and acetaminophen are the two best-known antifever medicines. Importantly, aspirin is not recommended for children with colds or flu, due to the possibility of Reye's syndrome, a very serious neurological condition that can even result in death. Although aspirin and acetaminophen can lower fever, their use is not necessary unless the fever is very high. A certain amount of body temperature elevation can help the body fight viruses more effectively. Therefore, we recommend that antifever medicines be used only when body temperature exceeds 103°F.

Decongestants

Decongestants are used to treat nasal and sinus congestion. They reduce the swelling of the mucous tissues. Decongestants are available in pill form, usually as pseudoephedrine, or in nose drops such as naphazoline, phenylephrine, and oxymetazoline. A high tolerance can quickly develop to nose drops; they become less effective with use. In fact, there can be a rebound effect; symptoms of congestion are known to get worse when use of nose drops is stopped.

Pseudoephedrine is a stimulant that constricts blood vessels in the nose and in many other parts of the body. This medicine should be avoided by those with high blood pressure, heart disease, or prostate enlargement, and by individuals who are currently on antidepressants or other stimulants. Also, decongestants can cause an increase in heart rate and can cause restlessness and anxiety. Using them past mid-afternoon can result in insomnia. We don't recommend the use of oral decongestants unless you have a severe case of nasal or sinus congestion.

Antihistamines

Antihistamines block the release of *histamine*—an inflammation-causing substance—from certain white blood cells. These drugs include diphenhydramine, chlorpheniramine, brompheniramine, and clemastine. They are best suited for treating allergies; we don't recommend the use of antihistamines for treating upper respiratory infections.

Many people take antihistamines at night when they have a cold or the flu, in order to sleep better. Most antihistamines are sedating and cause drowsiness. We prefer you use natural supplements for sleep, such as melatonin.

Pain Medicines

Pain medicines include aspirin, acetaminophen, naprosyn, and ibuprofen. As mentioned earlier, aspirin should be avoided in children who have colds or the flu, since it can cause a dangerous condition known as Reye's syndrome. Acetaminophen is fine when used occasionally, but regular use can cause liver or kidney damage. Similarly, naprosyn and ibuprofen can be used occasionally, but prolonged and regular intake can cause stomach upset, ulcers, and kidney damage. Both of these medicines work well for muscle aches and backache that accompany a bad case of the flu.

Cough Suppressants

Cough suppressants include codeine and dextromethorphan. Codeine is by prescription only and is very effective, except that it can cause nausea and allergic symptoms. (It is often used as a pain killer.) Dextromethorphan, the best-known nonprescription cough suppressant, is only mildly effective. Furthermore, studies in chick embryos found that dextromethorphan causes birth defects. Hence, women who are pregnant should avoid this drug. As a rule, coughing is your body's way to get rid of mucus and germs. So unless you have a severe cough or your cough is mostly dry, it is preferable not to use a cough suppressant.

Expectorants

Expectorants are medicines that loosen mucus. Guaifensin may be slightly effective in this regard. By loosening the mucus, it becomes easier to expel. Hydration—that is, keeping up with your fluid intake—is a very helpful and very safe natural way to loosen mucus. In Chapter 8, we discuss several other natural alternatives to conventional expectorants.

Sore-Throat Relief Medicines

Lozenges and sprays that numb the throat are partially effective. These sore-throat relief medicines include benzocaine, dyclonine, and phenol. They can provide temporary relief for a few minutes by deadening the nerve endings. If you have trouble swallowing food or trouble sleeping because of the pain, sore-throat relief medicines can temporarily help you.

RECENT DEVELOPMENTS WITH ANTIVIRAL DRUGS

Because of viruses' tiny size and their ability to mutate on a frequent basis, it has been more difficult for scientists to develop antiviral agents than it has been for them to develop antibacterial agents. But strides are being made. Over the past decade, scientists have developed a number of drugs that have antiviral activity against influenza, HIV, herpes, and other viruses. However, no effective antiviral agents are available to fight the rhinoviruses and adenoviruses that cause the common cold. Furthermore, many antiviral agents have side effects, and it would be counterproductive to take a drug that can cause side effects in order to treat such a benign condition as the common cold.

There are several antiviral agents that are partially effective against the flu virus. They may decrease the severity or length of the illness. The two best-known drugs in this category, amantadine and rimantadine, may reduce flu symptoms by about 50 percent. These prescription drugs are generally reserved for individuals who have chronic medical conditions that could become severely aggravated if the flu symptoms worsen. Both of these drugs have several side effects, including nausea, loss of appetite, nervousness, and lightheadedness.

New drugs are being developed that block the attachment of the cold virus to the mucous membranes of the upper respiratory system. One such drug is currently known as BIRR 4. This drug mimics a part of *intracellular adhesion molecule 1 (ICAM-1)*. Most cold viruses must attach to ICAM-1 in order to infect a human cell. The virus attaches to the BIRR 4 instead of to the ICAM-1 and, therefore, the virus does not act on the body. Considering such strides in medicine, new drugs that fight the flu or the common cold are likely to be developed in the future.

FACTS ON FLU VACCINES

Conventional treatment for the flu includes bed rest, plenty of fluids, pain medicines for the muscle aches, and cough suppressants. And there's another option. As discussed in Chapter 1, at the beginning of each flu season, the Vaccines and Related Biological Products Advisory

Committee of the Food and Drug Administration reviews the mutations that have occurred in the flu virus. They then make recommendations regarding which types of flu strains the vaccine for the upcoming flu season should include. Then a new vaccine is formulated.

It is important to realize that vaccines cannot protect against all of the mutations of the flu virus. Many people have the misconception that once they get the shot, they are immune for the rest of the year. The influenza virus vaccine provides partial immunity (about 80-percent efficacy) for a few months to a year, and adequate immunity is achieved two weeks after the vaccine is received. Side effects from the vaccine include tenderness, redness, and swelling at the site of the injection. Occasionally, muscle aches and fever can occur.

Flu vaccines are often given in October and November, and are most often recommended for the elderly, those with chronic heart or lung conditions, and certain health-care workers. For the time being, we do not recommend the vaccines for otherwise healthy individuals who have no risk factors. Some people experience fatigue, flu-like symptoms, and malaise after receiving the flu shot.

These vaccines are currently given by injection. However, it is possible that vaccine nasal sprays could someday be the standard method of administration. In a preliminary study funded by the National Institute of Allergy and Infectious Diseases, administration of an intranasal flu vaccine has been effective in preventing the flu virus in children (Belshe, 1998). But this is a preliminary finding, and continued research is needed.

DECIDING FACTORS FOR SEEING A DOCTOR

Both you and your doctor maintain hectic schedules. Neither of you want to book an appointment for minor, self-manageable symptoms. However, it is important to recognize symptoms indicating that something more serious is about to occur. Hence, we recommend the following guidelines in helping you decide when to seek medical attention.

If you have mild upper respiratory symptoms, such as a sore throat, runny nose, mild cough, and low-grade fever, it's best you first try the natural approaches discussed in this book (in Chapters 3 through 8). However, if you find that your symptoms are not improving, you should contact your doctor. The following is a short list of symptoms and signs that indicate a turn for the worse. For a more extended list, see "When Should I Call A Doctor?", pages 131 to 132.

- Your fever exceeds 102°F.

- You have severe nausea, have vomited, and can't keep fluids in.

- The mild headache has progressed to a moderate or severe headache.

- You have difficulty breathing.

- The mucus has turned thick yellow or green.

- You have a moderate to severe earache.

- You feel disoriented.

We recommend that you contact your doctor sooner if you are diabetic, have a chronic medical condition, already have poor lung function, or if the family member with these symptoms is an infant or a young child. Since children sometimes do not or cannot vocalize their symptoms, parents have to look out for potentially serious signs. These include high fever, avoidance of food or fluids, and lethargy.

Antibiotics are appropriate to prescribe when a doctor observes that a patient's symptoms may not simply be due to the common cold, that there is now indication that a bacterial infection has set in. The choice of the antibiotic depends on where the new infection has surfaced—for instance, in the ears, sinuses, or lungs. Serious upper respiratory tract symptoms to watch out for include drooling and the inability to swallow. These could be symptoms of tonsillitis, epiglottitis, or an abscess behind the pharynx, all of which require immediate medical attention.

Serious lower respiratory tract symptoms to look for include wheezing and shortness of breath. These could be signs of pneumonia, bronchitis, or asthma. Severe headache, often described as "my worst headache ever," along with a stiff neck, disorientation, and altered mental state, can be caused by meningitis, a complication of sinusitis, or other serious conditions.

THE PERSISTENT COUGH

Once the cold or the flu resolves, certain symptoms may continue and may annoy you for additional days and weeks. One particular symptom that is known to persist, particularly in individuals with the flu, is a dry cough. This is often due to damage or irritation that has occurred in the lungs, particularly in the bronchial tubes. We are not aware of natural herbs or supplements that can dramatically alleviate this problem, although there are several herbs that can provide a measure of relief (see Chapters 6 and 8). Sometimes a short course of prednisone for five to seven days can correct this problem. Prednisone is a synthetic steroid the blocks inappropriate irritation in the bronchi.

CONCLUSION

Antibiotics are prescribed to more than 50 percent of patients with the common cold. Ninety percent of these cases are due to viruses that do not respond to antibiotics.

When It's Not the Common Cold

It is important to know the warning signs of a serious progression of a respiratory infection, and also of allergies that can be mistaken for infections. Thus you can better manage your illness and, in many cases, avoid serious repercussions. So listed below are several explanations that will help you identify whether your symptoms are due to just a cold or to something more dangerous.

Allergy of the nose: involves itchiness of the nose, eyes, and throat, with no fever. The mucus from the nose is clear. An allergy is an inappropriate reaction (an overreaction) of the immune system.

Bronchitis: caused by inflammation of the bronchi, or the tubes that lead from the trachea to the lungs. Symptoms include cough and wheezing, along with a slight shortness of breath.

Influenza: a viral illness. Symptoms are similar to a cold, but are usually more severe. Fever is higher and muscle aches, headache, cough, and sore throat are more intense.

Otitis media: infection of the middle ear causing pain and a decrease in hearing. A visual exam of the ear with an otoscope reveals bulging and redness.

Pneumonia: usually includes a high fever accompanied by the production of large amounts of yellow or green mucus, high fever, cough, and chest pain. Pneumonias are most often bacterial.

Sinusitis: often involves a feeling of fullness in the face, pain in the upper jaw, and nasal discharge that is particularly thick yellow or green. There may or may not be fever and congestion.

Streptococcal pharyngitis: commonly known as strep throat. Symptoms are often similar to a cold and it's difficult for doctors to clinically distinguish between the two. However, patients with strep throat often have swelling in the lymph glands in the neck, a higher fever, and more severe tonsillitis, not the typical runny nose of a common cold. A throat culture often identifies the bug causing the strep throat.

Fortunately, doctors no longer have to rely on pulling out their prescription pads in order to appease patients. There are a number of effective natural supplements that can prevent or reduce the symptoms of colds and the flu. These supplements are far more effective than many over-the-counter drugs. The proper use of these supplements will reduce the need for the millions of prescriptions written every year for antibiotics that, at best, have no effect on the cold virus and, at worst, can have serious side effects. The following chapters will explore these natural remedies.

3 Vitamin C— Gold Medal Infection Fighter

T he story of vitamin C begins with scurvy, the oldest known disease of vitamin deficiency. This disease starts out with symptoms as mild as fatigue and bleeding gums, but eventually leads to death if left untreated. Scurvy is caused by vitamin-C deficiency. In fact, another name for vitamin C, *ascorbic acid*, literally means "without scurvy." Since the early years of vitamin C studies devoted to understanding and preventing scurvy, research on this water-soluble vitamin has expanded considerably.

Vitamin C is now recognized for the essential role it plays in the formation and maintenance of collagen (a protein that forms connective tissues) and for its capacity as an antioxidant. Antioxidants disarm compounds called free radicals that, if left unchecked, damage tissues and increase the risk of cancer, heart disease, arthritis, premature aging, and other degenerative diseases. Since this vitamin is water soluble, it fights its battles in the watery areas of the body, such as the blood, lymph fluid, and the areas within and between cells.

When it comes to the fight against colds and flus, vitamin C deserves a gold medal. Linus Pauling, Ph.D., a two-time Nobel laureate (chemistry in 1954 and peace in 1962), first sent vitamin C to the infection frontlines in his 1970s book, *Vitamin C and the Common Cold*. In this text, Pauling claimed that high doses of vitamin C could battle a cold. This claim sparked quite a firefight within the research community, with researchers devoted to either vindicating or vilifying vitamin C in this role. Now that the dust has settled, there is good evidence that vitamin C can play a part in decreasing symptoms of a cold. This chapter will explore the development of research regarding vitamin C's role in fighting the common cold, as well as the appropriate dosage and possible side effects.

THE COMMON COLD

Between 1930 and 1960, vitamin C was pigeonholed as a vitamin whose only function was to prevent scurvy, even though a few scientists already voiced their suspicions that vitamin C had immune-enhancing effects in general and, more specifically, an effect on the common cold. Soon after Pauling's book on vitamin C and the common cold was released, he published a scientific paper reanalyzing four of the best scientifically controlled vitamin C/cold experiments then available. This study supported his claims for vitamin-C benefits when used in amounts greater than 1 gram daily. Unfortunately, the next clinical trial to examine vitamin C found a beneficial effect but claimed that a breakdown of the rigorous scientific controls invalidated the results. Interest then waned for the potential connection between vitamin C and cold treatment.

Long-time vitamin-C researcher Harri Hemilä, Ph.D., from the Department of Public Health, University of Helsinki, Finland, has this to say about the resistance of the scientific community to vitamin C: "The general belief in conventional medical circles that vitamin C has no effect on the common cold seems surprising since essentially all of the placebo-controlled studies carried out both before and after Pauling's conclusion have shown a beneficial effect" (Hemilä, 1995). In fact, Hemilä himself conducted an exhaustive review of the research conducted between 1971 and 1992 (Hemilä, 1994). Only studies that compared 1 gram or greater of vitamin C with a placebo were included in his review, since smaller amounts of vitamin C are generally regarded as less effective for cold treatment. Although vitamin C wasn't shown to have a significant effect on the *incidence* of the common cold, taking 1 to 8 grams (in divided doses throughout the day) at the *onset* of a cold did reduce the cold's duration and severity. These benefits were seen in each of the twenty-one studies reviewed by Hemilä.

From the various studies included in this review, it was found that vitamin C decreased the duration and severity of cold symptoms by 5 to 35 percent, with the average improvement being 23 percent. When the studies were examined according to the amount of vitamin C taken by cold sufferers, studies providing 1 gram daily led to a 9-percent decrease in severity, while those based on 2 to 4 grams daily jumped up to a 29 percent decrease in severity. When looking at duration of symptoms, higher doses also produced better results. Clearly, vitamin C has a dose-dependent effect, meaning that the greater the dose of vitamin C taken, the stronger the effect. In summary, the scientific evidence indicates that the proper dosage and timing of vitamin C shortens the length of illness and reduces the symptoms of the common cold.

Even though the Hemilä review did not show a significant connection between vitamin C and the *prevention* of the common cold, subsequent research (including that from Hemilä himself) continues to revisit this issue. When Hemilä reviewed another set of studies involving 5,000 cold episodes, he reported that vitamin C does in fact result in a "30% decrease in the number of common cold episodes" (Hemilä, 1997). But this cold prevention effect is not seen across the board. It appears that vitamin C's role in preventing colds is limited to individuals under physical stress and to those who usually have a low dietary intake of the vitamin. (In contrast, vitamin C helps many people once a virus has *entered* the body.) For example, the cold-preventing effects were studied in a group of people with diets low in vitamin C. When these people supplemented with 1 gram or more, they had a 30-percent reduction in contracting colds, and a 46-percent decrease in recurrent infections.

Again, the only clinical trials included in this Hemilä review were those using more than 1 gram of vitamin C per day, since it may be difficult to statistically track the benefit of lesser supplement intakes. Although there was no difference in cold incidence between vitamin-C users and those taking a placebo in the data pooled for this study, patterns did emerge. Hemilä notes that "chest colds" and "throat colds" were less likely to develop in those taking vitamin C, even though "simple colds" were not affected by the vitamin. Despite the promising studies in support of vitamin C, skeptical researchers continue to suggest that the placebo effect is responsible for any beneficial results in studies.

STRESS

Both emotional and physical stress increase dietary needs for vitamin C, in order to maintain normal levels of vitamin C in the blood. The adrenal and pituitary glands (the "stress" glands) are major storage sites of vitamin C, and they can become depleted of this vitamin during times of stress. Therefore, the unique benefit of vitamin C for people under physical stress, reported by Hemilä, is not surprising.

The connection between stress and vitamin C is confirmed by further research focused on individuals experiencing physical stress. Studies involving military troops undergoing training, athletes participating in a marathon race, and children at a skiing camp in the Swiss Alps all found a considerable reduction in the incidence of the common cold for those supplementing with vitamin C (Hemilä, 1996). For example, the runners taking just 600 milligrams of vitamin C experienced fewer than half as many colds as those taking a placebo.

HEALTHY IMMUNE FUNCTION

Vitamin C is not known to clearly interact with invading cold germs. Rather, it has a general immune-boosting effect; in other words, it helps your body protect itself. For starters, because one of vitamin C's most basic roles in the body is to create collagen, which is needed to form and maintain body tissues, plenty of vitamin C maintains the strength of the body's physical barriers to infectious invaders.

Vitamin C also strengthens the immune system by increasing the production and activity of white blood cells, which are responsible for destroying foreign invaders such as viruses and bacteria. There is a reduction in white blood cell formation when vitamin C is deficient in the diet. In addition, vitamin C boosts production of interferon. Interferon consists of groups of glycoproteins that increase resistance to viruses and prevent them from replicating. Thus, the body's resistance to infection and disease improves when vitamin C intake is increased.

Certain immune system cells harness free radicals as ammunition in the fight against infection. Unfortunately, once the free radicals are released, they can inadvertently damage other immune system cells. As an antioxidant, vitamin C mops up any leftover free radicals.

THE FLU AND OTHER INFECTIONS

Although there are far fewer studies examining the effects of vitamin C on the flu than on vitamin C and the common cold, it makes sense that the overall immune-boosting effect of vitamin C would help people who have the flu. Research in animals indicates that the influenza virus decreases concentrations of vitamin C, although the specific effect of this on the course of disease is unknown (Hennet, 1992). However, limited and preliminary research has suggested that vitamin C helps prevent flu infections during the flu season (Sapozhnikov, 1976). More research is needed in this regard.

The common cold is not the only respiratory infection that vitamin C benefits; this vitamin seems to have an affinity for supporting healthy lungs. A group of older patients with bronchitis were enrolled in a study to compare the intake of 200 milligrams of vitamin C with the use of a placebo (Hunt, 1994). Those taking vitamin-C supplements fared significantly better than the placebo group in recovery from bronchitis.

The story is pretty similar with pneumonia. A review of the research involving this disease found that supplements of vitamin C led to more than 80-percent lower incidence of pneumonia (Hemilä, 1997). This is all the more impressive considering that these trials were based on very small amounts of vitamin C: 50 to 300 milligrams per day.

Asthma, although not an infectious disease itself, can be worsened by the presence of a respiratory infection. Similarly, exercise can also trigger asthma attacks and, for this reason, an asthmatic's tolerance for exercise is a useful measurement of asthma control. Twenty young asthmatics (ages seven to twenty-eight) suspended their use of regular asthma medications and instead took 2 grams of vitamin C or a placebo one hour before engaging in seven minutes of exercise on a treadmill (Cohen, 1997). This single large dose of vitamin C prevented a flare-up of asthma in 45 percent of the asthmatics, and lessened the severity of the attack in another 10 percent. Those who responded to the vitamin C coughed less and had less lung discomfort after exercise. As a follow-up, five of the asthmatics who responded positively to the vitamin C continued to take 500 milligrams of vitamin C daily for two weeks, and this supplementation continued to show a protective effect.

JUSTIFICATION FOR HIGHER INTAKE

Humans are one of only a handful of species who cannot produce their own vitamin C. Consequently, we depend on a continual dietary source of this vitamin. Although as little daily vitamin C as that found in a few orange slices prevents scurvy, amounts much larger than this appear to optimize immune function and overall health. But what is the optimal intake of vitamin C? There are different ways to try to answer this question.

The Recommended Dietary Allowance (RDA) for vitamin C is 60 milligrams daily. Is more better? A study published in the *American Journal of Clinical Nutrition* reports that large doses of ingested vitamin C may be excreted without being utilized (Blanchard, 1997). When a group of healthy men consumed vitamin C in increasing amounts from 200 milligrams to 2,500 milligrams per day, their serum levels increased only negligibly. James Blanchard, Ph.D., a professor of pharmacological sciences at the University of Arizona in Tucson, believes that the blood levels of vitamin C generally reflect the tissue levels. In other words, taking more than 200 milligrams on a daily basis may not raise body levels that much more, and the remainder will be excreted. However, much higher amounts than 60 milligrams may be needed to gain the most benefit during a cold infection—for example, 1 to 5 grams daily (which is the same as 1,000 to 5,000 milligrams).

As mentioned previously, the RDA for vitamin C is geared toward preventing scurvy. Some scientists believe that it should be raised to better reflect the anti-infection roles of vitamin C. According to Mark Levine, M.D., Ph.D., from the National Institutes of Health in Bethesda, Maryland, the RDA for vitamin C should triple to about 200 milligrams daily (Levine, 1996).

Although our Paleolithic ancestors probably consumed much more than our RDA for vitamin C daily, many modern people obtain far less through their diets of over-processed foods. Individuals who incorporate plenty of fruits and vegetables in their diets might consume 200 milligrams of vitamin C daily, but any diet would be hard-pressed to supply more than 500 milligrams daily. For this reason, supplemental sources of vitamin C are important for anyone wanting to consume a higher intake.

The segments of the population most at risk for low vitamin-C levels include alcoholics, elderly people in hospitals and nursing homes, and, surprisingly enough, young adults. When the diets and blood levels of vitamin C were tracked in a group of 232 college students, outright vitamin-C deficiency was only found in 1 to 2 percent of these students (Johnston, 1998). Yet 12 to 16 percent of them had marginal vitamin-C status, which can leave them at greater risk for infections.

Vitamin-C requirements increase beyond the RDA during times of stress (as discussed earlier in this chapter), fever, infection, burns, surgery, kidney and liver disease, gastrointestinal disturbance, cancer, oral contraceptive use, and alcohol or tobacco abuse. Cigarette smokers tend to have poor vitamin-C status, possibly as a result of the increased demand placed on this vitamin in neutralizing the numerous free radicals in cigarette smoke. The RDA has reflected the increased vitamin-C needs of smokers by raising requirements for this group to 100 milligrams daily. Some researchers recommend that smokers increase their intake of vitamin C even further, to at least 200 milligrams and perhaps up to 1,000 milligrams daily, in order to maintain adequate antioxidant protection. Individuals exposed to second-hand smoke may also require increased vitamin-C intake.

The optimal daily intake of vitamin C has not yet been determined, nor is it likely to be determined soon. Still, it seems clear that the RDA for vitamin C is too low, especially for certain segments of the population and also for those at risk during the cold season (and that's pretty much all of us).

DOSAGES AND FORMS

You don't have to wait until the sneezing starts to take vitamin C. Regular use of this vitamin—that is, taking 100 to 250 milligrams once or twice daily—keeps the immune system running strong. This range is a safe amount for most people to take on a long-term, year-round basis. (See pages 43 to 44 for the few exceptions.) And if you start noticing symptoms of a cold or flu, immediately take 3 to 5 grams of vitamin C. Then take another gram every two to three hours thereafter. If your stools start to loosen, cut back on intake.

Vitamin C is available in a wide variety of supplements, from multivitamins to stand-alone vitamin-C tablets, capsules, powders, drinks, and chewables. In fact, vitamin C is the most commonly available single supplement, usually found in doses of 500 milligrams. But vitamin C can be found in supplements ranging from 100 to 1,000 milligrams.

Foods rich in vitamin C can go a long way in optimizing vitamin-C intake. Supplementation should never be a substitute for a diet including plenty of fresh fruits and vegetables, especially since these foods provide hundreds of beneficial carotenoids and flavonoids that may enhance the functions of vitamin C. Excellent sources of vitamin C are: oranges and other citrus fruits; berries; green pepper; parsley; brussels sprouts; broccoli; collard greens; cantaloupe; and tomato juice. Good sources are: asparagus; green peas; potatoes; pineapples; corn; and bananas.

We are not aware of any studies that definitively confirm significant advantages of the natural form of vitamin C over the synthetic form. We do not recommend the use of chewable forms of vitamin C unless you brush your teeth immediately after. The acidity of the chewable tablets can be detrimental to tooth enamel.

TIMING IS EVERYTHING

Consuming adequate amounts of vitamin C (through food sources and possibly daily supplementation) year-round is sound advice for anyone. However, during the high-risk times of the cold and flu season, or when a cold actually strikes, you'll want to pay special attention to your vitamin-C intake. Furthermore, you'll want to increase intake considerably if you notice symptoms starting to begin.

One study found that when supplementation was started within twenty-four hours of symptoms, 6 grams of vitamin C for five days shortened colds by 48 percent (Asfora, 1977). Quite differently, starting twenty-four to forty-eight hours after the first symptoms only shortened the colds by 29 percent. When the vitamin-C regimen was started even later, no benefit was seen. In other words, the sooner you start increasing vitamin-C intake, the better.

For more than a decade, Dr. Sahelian has recommended vitamin C to thousands of patients with colds. His own clinical observations also indicate that timing is crucial. Some of the earliest symptoms of a cold are a strange or burning feeling in the nose and a slight soreness or uneasiness in the throat. The longer you wait, the less effective the therapy; even waiting two or three hours can make a difference. In fact, according to Dr. Sahelian's clinical experience, benefits from vitamin C are minimal after sixteen to twenty-four hours of the onset of the earliest cold symptoms. Once the full-blown symptoms start, vitamin C will make little or no difference.

SAFETY ISSUES AND CONCERNS

Excesses of vitamin C, a water-soluble vitamin, are excreted in the urine and thus do not accumulate to dangerous levels. Vitamin-C intakes of ten times or more of the RDA are very common in the United States and are not generally associated with any symptoms of toxicity. Several reviews of vitamin safety report that even prolonged, high intakes of vitamin C, exceeding a hundred times the RDA, are generally safe.

However, there is one small concern. One isolated study warns that vitamin C, in high doses, may have a harmful effect in addition to its beneficial effects. Dr. Podmore and colleagues at the University of Leicester found greater damage to DNA (according to certain markers) when a group of thirty healthy volunteers took 500 milligrams of vitamin C daily for six weeks (Podmore, 1998). However, the results of this study are difficult to interpret, as this amount of vitamin C also showed beneficial antioxidant effects in protecting DNA from damage. In other words, high doses of vitamin C both protected and hurt the DNA in cells. Although this report is generally inconsistent with much of the previous data on vitamin C, it may be prudent to limit long-term, daily intake of supplemental vitamin C to 500 milligrams until more information is available. However, higher dosages are appropriate for short-term treatment of the common cold.

Vitamin C does increase the absorption of iron. This is a beneficial effect for most people. But for individuals with certain conditions that interfere with the regulation of iron metabolism, such as hemochromatosis, an iron-absorption boost can be undesirable. Also, very high intakes of vitamin C can deplete the body of copper. The amount of copper found in many multivitamin/mineral supplements is adequate to prevent this problem. Also, the evidence is contradictory as to whether vitamin C accelerates the formation of urinary stones. This is a concern only if you are taking several grams of vitamin C daily for many years.

The most common side effect reported to result from very high vitamin-C intakes is gastrointestinal upset—namely nausea and diarrhea. You may want to experiment with what level of intake is tolerable for you. If you notice that your stools are loose, return to a lower dose.

CONCLUSION

During the cold season, and at any time of the year, supplemental vitamin-C intakes of 100 to 250 milligrams, once or twice daily, support a healthy immune system. However, this amount probably doesn't make the grade when your body is fighting a cold. We recommend immediately taking 3 to 5 grams of vitamin C when you first notice a cold coming on, and then take another gram every two to three hours thereafter. Scale back your vitamin-C intake if you experience any gastrointestinal upset.

There is good evidence that vitamin C is helpful in reducing the symptoms and length of cold episodes, if the timing is right. In many cases, vitamin C taken at the earliest onset of cold symptoms can either completely halt the progression of a cold or reduce the severity. Although this natural therapy may not help everyone avoid catching a cold—people under stress appear to gain the most protection in this department—vitamin C certainly deserves a prominent place in your medicine cabinet during the cold season. Its benefits are accentuated when combined with zinc lozenges and other supplements.

4

Zinc—A Cold's Worst Enemy

Your throat feels like sandpaper, your sneezes come in clusters, and your nose is raw from blowing. You pop a lozenge and allow it to dissolve in the back of your mouth. A couple of hours later your upper respiratory system is much happier. How can this be? That lozenge was a zinc lozenge. And if you continue to pop one every few hours, chances are good that you'll send your cold packing in half the time it would have lasted untreated. Zinc lozenges are truly the best option we currently have available as a common cold cure.

This chapter will explore the discovery and subsequent research regarding the use of zinc lozenges as a cold treatment, as well as the mechanisms by which zinc works. Detailed information is provided on how to incorporate zinc lozenges and zinc pills into your cold prevention and treatment plan.

EVIDENCE ON ZINC'S EFFECTIVENESS

Although it has been known since the 1940s that dietary zinc plays a general role in immune function, it wasn't until a serendipitous observation in 1979 that zinc lozenges were linked to the treatment of the common cold. There was a young girl who was under treatment for leukemia. She was being given zinc tablets for general immune-boosting purposes. One day she refused to swallow a zinc tablet. Instead, the little girl allowed the tablet to dissolve in her mouth. Her immune system was weakened by chemotherapy treatment, and the girl suffered from frequent colds. She was just developing another cold when this incident occurred. The burgeoning cold symptoms were relieved within mere hours of sucking on this makeshift zinc lozenge, leading to the hypothesis that the zinc lozenge was responsible for her cold relief. Incidentally, the girl later recovered from her other health problems.

Following this initial discovery, clinical trials were proposed to formally examine the potential of zinc lozenges as a treatment for colds. The first clinical trial to take a closer look was published in the mid-1980s (Eby, 1984). Volunteers with colds from the community of Austin, Texas were either assigned to a group taking zinc (in the form of zinc gluconate) lozenges or dummy lozenges (placebos). A seven-day supply was allotted to each of the 120 cold sufferers. The participants of the first group each took two lozenges (one right after the other) as a loading dose, and then a lozenge dissolved in the mouth every two hours. Within twenty-four hours of starting this regimen, 22 percent of those who were actually using the zinc lozenges reported a complete resolution of their cold symptoms. Not one participant taking the dummy lozenges could say the same. And by the end of the week, 90 percent of the zinc group had kicked their colds, while only 49 percent of the placebo group were cold-free. Results showed that the zinc group averaged cold symptoms for about four days, while the placebo group's colds stuck around for a miserable eleven days.

Of course, scientists are never satisfied with just one study. So it wasn't long before follow-up work was underway. A 1992 study of seventy-three young adults showed similar results as the first study, namely that people sucking on zinc lozenges recovered from their colds in an average of 4.3 days, while those taking the placebo lozenges endured their colds for 9.2 days (Godfrey, 1992). The symptoms that seemed to be most susceptible to the zinc lozenges were cough, runny nose, and sinus congestion.

An even stronger case for the power of zinc lozenges was established when a 1996 study was published in the well-respected journal *Annals of Internal Medicine.* Sherif Mossad, M.D., and colleagues at the Cleveland Clinic Foundation enrolled 100 men and women into their study. The participants had all developed symptoms consistent with a cold within the past twenty-four hours. Half were given a supply of lemon-flavored zinc lozenges containing 13.3 milligrams of zinc (in the zinc gluconate form). They were instructed to let one lozenge dissolve in their mouths every two hours while awake, and to continue this regimen for the duration of their illness. The other half unknowingly received a supply of dummy lozenges developed to have a medicinal taste similar to the zinc lozenges.

All of the subjects recorded their symptoms—cough, headache, hoarseness, muscle ache, nasal drainage, nasal congestion, scratchy or sore throat, sneezing, and fever—and how long each symptom lasted. According to Dr. Mossad, "the time to complete resolution of symptoms was significantly shorter in the zinc group than in the placebo group (median, 4.4 days compared with 7.6 days . . .)." In particular, the zinc-lozenge-takers recorded fewer days of coughing, headaches, hoarseness, stuffy nose, nasal drainage, and sore throat. The zinc lozenges provided much welcomed relief.

After reviewing the evidence regarding zinc lozenges in controlled trials, Dr. S. Marshall from Queen's University in Kingston, Ontario, Canada concludes that "evidence supports use of zinc gluconate lozenges for reducing the symptoms and duration of the common cold, but the side effects, bad taste, and therapeutic protocol might limit patient compliance" (Marshall, 1998). See pages 56 to 57 for more information on safety issues and concerns. And for information on children's use of zinc lozenges, see pages 118 to 119.

Dr. Sahelian's first personal experience with zinc lozenges was seven years ago. He had returned from a trip in France and the combination of the travel, inadequate sleep, and jet lag were too much for his immune system. Dr. Sahelian felt the beginnings of a sore throat and nasal congestion. On the way home from the airport, he stopped by a health food store and purchased a bottle of zinc lozenges. Within a few hours, the symptoms had disappeared. Over the years, zinc lozenges have several times more aborted the start of a cold for him. Based on personal and professional experience, reports from patients, and the scientific literature, Dr. Sahelian is convinced that zinc lozenges shorten the duration of cold symptoms.

Over the past few years, Dr. Sahelian has recommended zinc lozenges to hundreds of patients. The majority of these patients appreciate the reduction in symptoms that zinc lozenges provide. They feel better, do not need to rely as much on pharmaceutical medicines, and are able to return to work much more quickly. The doctor finds zinc to be most effective when taken within hours of onset of the earliest symptoms of a cold. However, even if the zinc lozenges are started after the first twenty-four hours, they still provide benefits. The two most frequent complaints are nausea and unpleasant taste.

HOW ZINC WORKS

With several positive studies under zinc's belt, the next obvious question is, "How do zinc lozenges successfully treat the common cold?" Researchers have been surprised, over the course of several studies, by reports from study participants that zinc lozenges bring symptom relief within a few minutes of popping a lozenge. Such a quick effect can't be accounted for by the virus-fighting ability of the zinc, which takes longer to act. Something else must be at work.

The "something else" is believed to be zinc's direct action on nerves in the face and nose. Think about what happens if you are just about to sneeze and you press your finger against your upper lip; the imminent sneeze is aborted. Obviously, zinc lozenges dissolved in the mouth can't be exactly like the physical pressure of a finger. But the reason that finger pressure can abort a sneeze attack is that it acts as a clamp to prevent the nerve transmission of the sneeze message to the brain. This same effect may also be achieved with zinc, albeit in a slightly different way (Novick, 1997).

The dissolving zinc lozenge releases ions of zinc that naturally enter the blood in the face and nasal area. This leads to a temporarily high concentration of zinc, which interferes with the nerve impulses for sneezing, as well as for nasal discharge and nasal congestion. This effect lasts until zinc levels drop down again to where they were at before supplementation. It appears to take between one to three hours for this effect to wear off, which, not surprisingly, is about the frequency scientific studies suggest for taking zinc lozenges—that is, every two hours.

Another explanation for the relief experienced by cold sufferers who are taking zinc is a more direct antiviral effect. Viruses, as explained in Chapter 1, enter your cells and turn them into virus-making factories. To get into the cells, viruses use various mechanisms. For example, the rhinovirus (which accounts for up to half of all colds) makes use of a substance called ICAM–1 (intercellular adhesion molecules) to attach to and enter into your cells. Anything that interferes with the connection between rhinovirus and ICAM–1 blocks the viral infection. It has been suggested that zinc does just that (Novick, 1996).

There are several additional mechanisms that could account for the effectiveness of zinc lozenges (Garland, 1998). Laboratory studies show that zinc affects a direct inhibition of cold viruses' abilities to reproduce themselves. Zinc does this by preventing the formation of proteins that are needed for viral replication and by strengthening cell membranes from viral attack. It has also been suggested that zinc boosts production of gamma interferon, which is a powerful antiviral substance produced by the immune system. In addition, the astringency of zinc helps to dry out nasal tissues and to quicken their healing.

WHY ZINC FAILED IN SOME STUDIES

Given the encouraging studies discussed above, it's hard to believe that there are several studies in which zinc failed to help cold sufferers. For example, one study comparing 23-milligram zinc lozenges (in the form zinc gluconate, with mannitol and sorbitol added for sweetness) with placebos in 110 cold patients found no benefit from the zinc when taken every two hours (Smith, 1989). Similarly, 10-milligram lozenges of zinc acetate used by sixty-three individuals were found to result in no significant difference when compared with placebo lozenges (Douglas, 1987). And a study using zinc gluconate lozenges that contained 4.5 milligrams of zinc also found that the zinc provided no benefit (Weismann, 1990).

Furthermore, the first study to examine the potential of zinc lozenges in children and teenagers didn't make the grade for cold treatment. This study assigned 249 students (grades one to twelve) to take either zinc lozenges or placebo lozenges (Macknin, 1998). Each zinc lozenge supplied 10 milligrams of zinc (in the zinc gluconate glycine form), and five to six lozenges were taken daily, starting within twenty-four hours of the first cold symptoms. There was no significant difference between groups concerning how many days the youths suffered from a variety of cold symptoms. However, more kids in the zinc group reported that the lozenges caused a bad taste, nausea, and mouth irritation. The researchers summed up, "[zinc] lozenges in the dosages studied were ineffective in relieving cold symptoms in children and adolescents in this . . . trial."

What could account for zinc's failure in these studies? There are some clues when each of these studies are examined individually. For starters, the Weismann study used zinc gluconate lozenges that provided only 4.5 milligrams of zinc per lozenge, whereas all of the studies showing good results used 13.3 to 23.0 milligrams of zinc. Quite simply, the amount of zinc in this study was probably inadequate. In addition, the Macknin study of zinc use for children only used a fraction of the amount of zinc generally used in studies applied to adults. So again, there may have been an issue of insufficient dosage. It is not known if the cold-busting effects of zinc can occur from lower doses for children, due to their the smaller size, or if they require the same amount as adults.

For the other failed studies, zinc-researcher George Eby (the father of the girl with leukemia discussed previously) thinks he may have an even better explanation (Eby, 1997). The form of zinc in the lozenge, as well as the absence or presence of other compounds in the lozenge, affects the ability of the body to access the zinc. Eby suggests that lozenges that release zinc ions that are the same pH (a measure of acidity) as the body are bioavailable (able to be absorbed and used by the body), whereas lozenges that release neutral or negatively charged zinc are not beneficial. Eby developed a scale of comparison for various zinc lozenge preparations; he dubbed this scale the *zinc ion availability* or *ZIA*.

Thus, Eby explains that it is not only the amount of zinc in a lozenge that determines its effect, but also the body's ability to capture the zinc ions. Zinc is not found in a pure form in lozenges; it can be bound to any of a number of other molecules to form zinc gluconate, zinc acetate, and many other complexes. These other molecules (that is, the gluconate, acetate, etc.) affect the absorption and use of zinc by the body. In addition, other substances added to lozenges for flavor or other reasons can also affect zinc availability. In short, all zinc lozenges are not similar.

Studies using zinc gluconate lozenges, each supplying 11.5 to 23.0 milligrams of zinc, were found to have higher ZIA scores and a corresponding therapeutic effect for the common cold. They lead to a 1.6- to 7.0-day decrease in the duration of symptoms. In addition, Eby reports that studies based on zinc lozenges with a near-zero ZIA score (including zinc orotate and zinc aspartate) found no effect, good or bad, for the zinc treatment. Meanwhile, studies with a negative ZIA score, which included the forms of zinc gluconate-citrate and zinc acetate-tartarate-carbonate, actually showed a lengthening of cold duration. Many more studies are certainly needed before we determine the ideal forms and dosages of zinc lozenges.

ZINC'S ESSENTIAL ROLE IN THE DIET

About 2 to 3 grams of zinc are found in the body at any one time. Since body-stores of zinc are not readily mobilized, a daily supply from the diet is necessary. Requirements for healthy adults range from 12 to 15 milligrams daily. If intake is low, the body can compensate in the short-term by absorbing a greater amount of dietary zinc and reducing zinc excretion. But over time, inadequate zinc intake takes its toll on the body.

Insufficient zinc affects a wide variety of bodily functions, and depressed immunity is one of the first signs. Specifically, a marginal zinc deficiency decreases the number of natural killer cells, while optimal zinc intake boosts levels of antibodies and increases numbers of T-lymphocytes (Ozturk, 1994). Other deficiency symptoms include changes in hair and nails, sterility, skin inflammation, lethargy, anemia, poor wound healing, and a loss of taste and smell. Zinc deficiency can also cause significant damage to the retina and impair nerve conductivity. Groups at increased risk of zinc deficiency are alcoholics and those with sickle cell anemia, chronic renal (kidney) disease, and other long-term debilitating diseases.

Zinc deficiencies may have reached epidemic proportions. As many as one in three Americans over age fifty is thought to have an undiagnosed marginal zinc deficiency. Surveys show that only 10 percent of Americans consume even the minimal recommended intake for zinc. The situation is getting worse, not better; average zinc intakes are lower than they were just a decade ago. Mild zinc deficiencies are difficult to detect. Many times, the first indication is an increased susceptibility to infections, although a deficiency may show itself as white spots on the fingernails. (Please note that there may be other nutritional causes of these white spots.)

Several circumstances can increase zinc requirements. For example, some studies show that zinc requirements increase during the last half of pregnancy, during and after an infection, and after frequent or excessive consumption of alcohol. In addition, stomach acid is important for proper absorption of zinc, so any condition or medication that lowers stomach acid may limit the availability of zinc.

Diet plays a role in zinc status. Many people are dramatically increasing their intake of fiber for health reasons, but they are inadvertently setting themselves up for a zinc deficiency because excess fiber blocks zinc absorption. In addition, since meat is a good dietary source of zinc, vegetarians may be at risk for zinc deficiency. Dietary sources of zinc include oysters, shrimp, red meat, poultry, organ meats (liver), pork, milk, and egg yolks. Moderate sources are whole grain breads and cereals, and wheat germ.

THE BEST DOSAGE AND FORM

Since deficiencies are sometimes difficult to diagnose, and moderate-dose supplements are generally safe, it makes sense for anyone at risk for low zinc levels to take a zinc supplement daily. It's convenient to take zinc as part of a multiple vitamin/mineral dietary supplement. A daily supplement providing about 10 to 15 milligrams of zinc is usually adequate to prevent deficiencies and to optimize immune function.

There are many forms of zinc that can be used in lozenges, but it just makes sense to follow the form and dosage that scientific research has found to be more consistent. Zinc gluconate or zinc gluconate/glycine lozenges, supplying 11.5 milligrams to 23.0 milligrams of zinc per lozenge, have shown the best results in the research. Anecdotal evidence also indicates that zinc acetate lozenges are effective.

Lozenges sweetened with fructose appear to retain effectiveness, but other ingredients in lozenges may interfere with treatment. Some researchers suggest avoiding lozenges that contain citric acid, since the citric acid, when dissolved in the saliva, does not allow the zinc ions to be released (Zarembo, 1992). Ascorbic acid, tartaric acid, mannitol, and sorbitol seem to have similar inhibiting effects (Garland, 1998). Certainly, more research is needed.

Since the nose and nasal passages are ground zero for most cold infections, some people have wondered if nose drops or nasal sprays containing zinc might be even more effective for cold treatment, in place of throat lozenges or supplement pills. Starting as far back as 1903, zinc applied to the nasal tissues has been used occasionally as a decongestant, but this decongestant effect seems to be the only benefit. Zinc used in this way does not have the same ability to shorten the length of the common cold as the lozenges do, for reasons that remain unclear (Eby, 1997). Another disadvantage is that nasal sprays need to be used very often (every ten to fifteen minutes), since substances are cleared very rapidly from the nose. Another downside is the potential for nasal discomfort and tissue irritation. All in all, the lozenges remain a better choice.

Swallowing zinc pills, as opposed to sucking on lozenges, is better suited to general immune enhancement. When taken as an oral supplement, zinc gluconate is among the best choices, as it is less irritating to the digestive system (one of the main complaints of zinc supplementation). Zinc citrate, zinc methionine, and zinc mono-methionine are also good choices if you choose to take a zinc supplement. But for the relief of cold symptoms, use lozenges and allow them to dissolve slowly in your mouth. Keep them in the mouth for as long as possible, as this will allow the throat tissue to be exposed to the zinc ions for a considerable duration.

TIMING IS EVERYTHING

In the twelve to twenty-four hours before the earliest symptoms of a cold emerge, the cold virus is replicating itself at breakneck speed. From here on, your immune defenses are playing a game of catch-up. This is why it is absolutely crucial to start using zinc lozenges when you have the first inkling that a cold might be brewing. In our personal experience, starting zinc lozenges within mere hours of the first cold symptom frequently aborts the cold, a full-fledged illness rarely takes hold. Research also bears this out. Study participants starting zinc-lozenge treatment on the second day of symptoms, as opposed to those starting within twenty-four hours, endured symptoms for a day and a half more than if they'd started right away (Garland, 1998).

In fact, the best plan is to keep zinc lozenges on hand so you'll be ready to pop one, be it in the middle of the night or in the middle of a busy workday. If that's not possible, make it your goal to start taking zinc lozenges within twelve to twenty-four hours of your first symptom. You'll want to suck on a lozenge every two to three hours while you are awake, and keep this up until your last symptom disappears.

SAFETY ISSUES AND CONCERNS

Zinc lozenges do have a few negative aspects. A number of people report that frequent use of lozenges makes them feel queasy and/or results in mouth irritation. Others simply dislike the metallic taste that some lozenges have. If you have one of these problems, you may want to experiment with different brands. And if you continue to have problems, you could turn your attention to other natural cold remedies discussed in this book. Mrs. Toews found that only certain brands irritate her mouth; other brands are completely tolerable. Another tip is to eat a small snack or drink something prior to popping a lozenge; this can prevent the nausea and vomiting associated with the lozenges (Eby, 1984).

Taking large amounts of zinc for short periods of time (that is, the week or so it takes to lick your cold) is generally harmless. However, long-term use (over several weeks or more) of zinc lozenges or oral supplements can cause problems. Specifically, continuous high zinc intake can interfere with copper absorption, resulting in a copper deficiency. Copper intake should be increased if zinc is used for extended periods. (The exception is people with Wilson's disease, a disorder in which copper accumulates in the body. Such people should *never* take copper.) Many supplement manufacturers recognize this problem and already include copper in their formulas. Take the time to check the label. If you are supplementing with copper, 1 to 3 milligrams is a prudent amount to take.

Ironically, taking too much zinc over long periods of time can actually result in impaired immune function (Schlesinger, 1993). However, the level this occurs at is quite high, in excess of 300 milligrams daily. Using lozenges for short periods to treat cold symptoms and supplementing with 5 to 15 milligrams of zinc daily as part of a multiple vitamin/mineral supplement is safe and beneficial.

CONCLUSION

A vigilant, well-running immune system depends on adequate amounts of zinc every day. Even a marginal deficiency of this mineral lowers your defenses against infection and disease. Keep an eye on your food choices to make sure you're getting plenty of dietary zinc, and consider a dietary supplement if your food choices don't provide adequate zinc, to keep your immune system running well. Supplementing with moderate amounts of zinc— about 15 milligrams daily—may improve immune function in zinc-deficient individuals.

When a cold hits, however, it's time to strike back with higher amounts of zinc, used on a short-term basis and in the form of lozenges. Don't let this year's crop of cold viruses catch you unprepared! Start taking zinc lozenges as soon as possible. Choose zinc gluconate, zinc gluconate/ glycine, or zinc acetate lozenges that supply 11.5 to 23.0 milligrams of zinc per lozenge. Your best bet is to allow a zinc lozenge to dissolve in the back of your mouth every two to three hours, while awake. Keep this up until your last symptom disappears. Keep the lozenge in your mouth for as long as possible before swallowing. The longer you keep them in your mouth, the better the chance the zinc has to kill the viruses in the throat and upper respiratory tract. You may need to use the lozenges less frequently if you find them irritating.

5 Echinacea— Herbal Immune Activator

Echinacea, an herb with a long-recognized role in fighting infections, is rapidly becoming a household word. And with good reason. Echinacea has been tested in a wide variety of chronic and acute infections, and the common cold and the flu is where this herb really stands out, especially when it is taken during the very early stages of illness.

Echinacea is useful once symptoms of a cold or flu develop—to keep your misery as brief as possible. This chapter will give you the full story on this helpful herb, from its history to its application.

ECHINACEA'S BOTANICAL BACKGROUND

Echinacea is also known as purple coneflower, an apt name considering its purple flower petals and protruding center. Other common names for echinacea include black sampson, red sunflower, and comb flower. There are nine species of this plant, but only three of them are in common usage as herbal healers: *Echinacea purpurea, E. angustifolia,* and *E. pallida.*

Echinacea grows extensively in the wild. It is especially plentiful in the plains areas of North America ranging from Texas to Canada. Most of the echinacea that finds its way into herbal teas and herbal formulas is cultivated and harvested expressly for this purpose. That's a good thing, since overharvesting a wild herb—especially of an herb that has a growing popularity—could deplete natural sources. Herb farms are located throughout the United States and in Europe.

Echinacea is made up of many different chemical constituents, and it is likely that several of these constituents work in synergy to evoke immune stimulation. The active components of echinacea can be divided into several categories: polysaccharides; caffeic acid derivatives; and alkylamides. Other constituents include flavonoids, glycoproteins, and polyacetylenes, whose effects in the body are not completely understood.

Polysaccharides

Several studies show that echinacea's polysaccharides, or complex sugar molecules, stimulate key immune system cells. One study extracted polysaccharides from *E. purpurea* and found that they activated phagocytes, the immune system cells that engulf and digest foreign invaders (Roesler, 1991). Similarly, another study found that polysaccharides from *E. purpurea* improved the activity of macrophages, immune cells that also engulf and digest other cells and foreign invaders (Steinmuller, 1993).

Caffeic Acid Derivatives

The unique caffeic acid derivative present in echinacea is echinacoside. This component is found in the highest concentrations in the roots, although it is also present to a lesser extent in echinacea flowers. Aside from echinacoside, there are several other caffeic acid derivatives that may have a role in the immune-boosting effect of echinacea (Combest, 1997).

Alkylamides

Alkylamides are concentrated primarily in the roots of the echinacea plant. They are responsible for the tingling or numbing sensation on the tongue when the herb is chewed or when liquid extracts are used. Herbalists have used the "tongue tingle" as an informal test to assess the quality of echinacea extracts (Perry, 1997). However, it is not known how effective this test is as a determinant of quality products.

ECHINACEA'S ILLUSTRIOUS HISTORY

As with most herbs, echinacea has a long history of traditional use. In fact, echinacea was one of the most widely used herbs in Native American medicine. It isn't known when Native Americans first began using echinacea as a medicinal herb, but it has been found in archaeological sites dating back to the seventeenth century. Medicinal use of echinacea is most firmly rooted with many of the plains tribes, which is not surprising since echinacea grows prolifically through the plains.

Echinacea's traditional applications are many and varied. It has been used to treat toothaches, sore throats, coughs, infections, snakebites, and colic (Combest, 1997). In most cases, the afflicted individual was instructed to suck or chew on the plant's root. Echinacea was also applied directly to venomous bites and other skin wounds.

Many Native American tribes shared their knowledge of echinacea with European colonists, as well as their uses of other herbs in their pharmacopoeia. The colonists were very receptive to this information, since it was difficult to bring conventional medicines over from Europe. Back in Europe, echinacea may have been known to botanists as early as the 1690s. However, it wasn't until 1794 that this herb received its European name of echinacea. The botanist Moench dubbed the genus Echinacea after the Greek word for sea urchin (*echinos*), which described the look of echinacea's protruding cone in the center of the flower.

Dr. H.F.C. Meyer, a physician from Pawnee City, Nebraska, was the first to popularize the medicinal use of echinacea (Tyler, 1993). In the 1870s, Dr. Meyer—who had learned of echinacea from local Native American tribes—created an echinacea formula using *E. angustifolia* and patented it as a medicine. The formula also contained other herbs, including hops and wormwood. This formula, called "Meyer's Blood Purifier," was recommended by Meyer for numerous maladies, including colds and flu. It gained a following and was popular for many years.

Dr. Meyer sent a sample of echinacea to two respected medical doctors, along with grandiose claims about the herb. He specifically claimed that it could cure snake bites. To prove it, Dr. Meyer told the doctors that he would allow himself to be bitten by a rattlesnake in their presence, and thereafter treat himself only with echinacea (Hobbs, 1990). The two doctors—John King and John Uri Lloyd, who were part of the Eclectic movement—declined his offer, chalking it up to hyperbole. The initial skepticism of King and Lloyd was transformed into respect for echinacea after they began to work with Meyer's herb sample.

From the mid-1800s through the 1930s, the Eclectic school of medicine was an influential branch of medical philosophy. Eclectic physicians relied in large part on herbs in their medical practice. King and Lloyd helped echinacea become one of the mainstay herbs of Eclectic medicine. In this regard, it was found useful in the treatment of many illnesses, namely infections such as diphtheria, typhoid, meningitis, and syphilis. It was also used to stimulate digestion and to heal insect and animal bites. In fact, at one point in the late 1800s, echinacea was the most prescribed herbal medicine due to its role in treating a wide range of infections. Eclectic physicians tended to use a high-alcohol liquid extract of echinacea.

The conventional medical establishment dismissed echinacea in the early part of the twentieth century. In fact, the *Journal of the American Medical Association* accused echinacea of being quackery. Despite its status as persona non grata to the medical establishment, many conventional physicians continued to use this herb. And, in partial redemption of its reputation, echinacea was included in the United States *National Formulary* from 1916 until it stopped being published in 1950.

Interest in echinacea waned through the early and middle decades of the twentieth century in the United States, due in large part to the discovery and reliance on antibiotics. However, research continued in Europe. Germany carried the torch by continuing to use and research echinacea, and even today echinacea is more widely used in Germany than in the United States. In the 1930s, when Dr. Gerhard Madaus, founder of a German pharmaceutical company, came to the United States to obtain seeds of the *E. angustifolia* plant, he inadvertently arrived home with *E. purpurea* seeds. As a result, much of the modern research has been conducted with the *E. purpurea* family of echinacea (Brown, 1996).

THE WAY ECHINACEA WORKS

Rather than having a direct germ-killing effect, echinacea's benefits are traced to the stimulation of the body's own immune defenses. In this way, echinacea helps the body protect itself against infectious invaders.

In terms of immune system enhancement, the value of echinacea's polysaccharides is backed by a large body of evidence. However, other components of echinacea are likely to perk up immune function, as well. When researchers examined various parts of the echinacea plant and various species of echinacea, they found that the immune system was buoyed by both the juice extracted from the upper parts of *E. purpurea*, as well as the roots of the *E. pallida*, *E. angustifolia*, and *E. purpurea* species (Bauer, 1996).

Echinacea increases the production of immune system cells that engage in phagocytosis—that is, the process of engulfing and digesting bacteria and other invaders. When mice are given alcohol extracts (tinctures) of echinacea root, their immune systems' phagocytes (such as macrophages) are stimulated (Bauer, 1988). In this study, the fat-soluble parts of the extract showed the strongest effect. More animal research confirms that echinacea increases the production of phagocytes in the body, and more phagocytes means that a virus has a lesser chance of continuing to infect the body (Roesler, 1991).

When echinacea is put to the test in a head-to-head challenge with microbes, it comes out ahead. In the laboratory, the *Candida albicans* fungus was mixed with immune system cells taken from human volunteers. The presence of echinacea increased the phagocytosis of the fungi by 30 to 45 percent (Wildfeuer, 1994). A similar study found that phagocytosis was even more effective when echinacea was combined with other plant extracts, specifically boneset, arnica, and wild indigo (Wagner, 1991). When humans are given echinacea and the phagocytic activity of the immune cells in their blood is studied, echinacea is found to significantly enhance this immune system parameter. Echinacea may also spur production of interferon, an immune system protein that prevents viral replication (Leuttig, 1989).

THE THEORY PUT INTO PRACTICE

Knowing echinacea's mechanisms of action is valuable, but the more important question in most people's minds is, "What happens when you have a cold and take echinacea?" Several studies have been conducted to answer this question.

A single-blind clinical trial randomly divided thirty-two cold sufferers into two groups. One group took a combination of echinacea extract and vitamin C (100 milligrams), while the other unknowingly took placebos (Scaglione, 1995). The effect of the echinacea / vitamin C combination was assessed by charting how long the illness lasted (in terms of the symptom of runny nose) and how many tissues were used each day. As it turned out, the placebo group reported cold symptoms for four days, while the echinacea group only reported cold symptoms for three days. The number of tissues used was also significantly more in the placebo group—1,168 compared with 882.

In another study, a multi-centered, uncontrolled trial—meaning that no placebo group was used—tracked the effects of echinacea in seventy-seven adults who had come down with upper respiratory infections (Degenring, 1995). In this study, an alcohol-based extract made from the stems, leaves, and roots of *E. purpurea* was utilized—thirty drops of the extract, three times daily for fourteen days. Study participants were excluded if their infection symptoms emerged more than three days before the start of echinacea treatment.

The infections were rated by a physician on the first day of research, as well as three more times over the course of the month-long study. A "symptoms index" that combined many symptoms (including fever, cough, sore throat, headache, and several others) was used to judge the efficacy of the echinacea treatment. This symptoms index combined the scores of each symptom into a single number; the higher the number, the more severe the infection.

The symptom scores dropped quickly during the fourteen days of echinacea use, with 72 percent of the participants becoming symptom-free by the end of the treatment period. According to the physician assessments, the echinacea was clinically relevant in 87 percent of the patients. The patients themselves rated the efficacy of the echinacea at 88 percent. Overall, the researchers of this study concluded that echinacea ". . . can be employed with a very good chance of success in the prophylaxis [or prevention] and treatment of recurrent infections."

Another study investigated how a liquid extract of *E. purpurea* influenced the duration and severity of cold infections (Schoenberger, 1992). Half of the 108 participants took echinacea extract, while the other half were given placebos. Although this study lasted only eight weeks, the researchers reported that the members of the group taking echinacea were less likely to become infected, and if they did develop a cold, the individuals in this group had less severe symptoms and recovered more quickly.

However, in one study, echinacea was *not* confirmed to prevent upper respiratory tract infections (Melchart, 1998). In this double-blind clinical trial, the results showed that echinacea was only slightly more effective than the placebo in preventing colds. Yet despite the fact that the participants did not know whether they were in the real or fake supplement groups, it is intriguing that those who actually took the echinacea reported that they felt this herb to be helpful.

In regards to the flu, the clinical research is limited. However, there is a study that tracked the potential benefits of echinacea in 180 individuals suffering from influenza infection (Braunig, 1992). These people were assigned to one of three groups: placebo; 450 milligrams per day of echinacea; or 900 milligrams per day of echinacea. The lower amount of echinacea did not yield impressive results. However, the group taking 900 milligrams of echinacea daily had a significant improvement of flu symptoms, including reduced fatigue, chills, sore throat, muscle aches, and headaches.

THE BEST DOSAGE AND FORM

Although there are nine species of echinacea—and three of these are commonly used in herbal formulas—there is no definitive answer, at this time, as to which species of echinacea is best for boosting immune function. To cover your bases, you might want to choose an echinacea supplement that combines two or more of the species. Moreover, it has not yet been definitively established which part of the plant (root, flowers, stems, or leaves) is preferable to use. In short, more research is needed to answer these practical questions. Until then, you can take comfort in the fact that echinacea, regardless of the species or parts used, has consistently shown itself to be effective in revving up the immune system to better fight off respiratory infections.

Despite being an herb native to North America, echinacea has an even stronger following in Europe, where both the oral and injectable forms are available. But in the United States, oral forms—taken as the fresh or dried herb, ground or powdered, in capsules, tablets, as tincture, or made into teas or other beverages—are used exclusively, since the injectable form is not available. Of these forms, there is some debate as to whether the liquid form of echinacea might be preferable. It has been suggested that this form triggers an immune response by stimulating lymphatic tissue in the mouth (Tyler, 1993). If true, then the liquid extracts would be a better form to use than capsules containing powdered echinacea. However, we have no solid information regarding this issue and there are even suggestions that the opposite is true—that the powdered extracts may be better since they are more concentrated and have a longer shelf life.

Herbalist Christopher Hobbs cuts through these arguments to make the following point: "The form (powder, liquid, etc.) is less important than the quality of the starting herb and the care taken in the manufacturing process, though most, if not all, of the clinical and laboratory tests and reports used a liquid alcoholic preparation" (Hobbs, 1994). We tend to agree with this viewpoint. However, it makes sense to choose the form that you are personally the most comfortable with and are the most likely to use. For example, if you are traveling, it is unlikely that you'll have the time or equipment to brew several cups of echinacea tea daily. In such a case, the tincture or capsule form might be more appropriate.

About 1 teaspoon of the dried root is used to brew 1 cup of tea, and you should drink several cups of this tea daily during an acute infection. As an added benefit, the warm tea is soothing to a sore throat. When using echinacea as an alcohol-, water-, or glycerin-based extract, take 1 to 2 milliliters, three times daily. Tinctures—concentrated fluid extracts of herbs—can be used in the amount of 3 to 4 milliliters, three times daily. If you are taking echinacea caplets, you'll want to take 600 to 1,200 milligrams, split into three to four doses throughout the day. You can continue taking echinacea, in whatever form you prefer, until your symptoms start to improve. For the majority of the cases, echinacea use won't exceed two weeks.

A growing number of supplements designed to support immune function and treat colds and the flu contain echinacea. Among the more common formulas are echinacea with vitamin C and echinacea with goldenseal. Scientific support for specific combinations is lacking, but there is a theoretical basis for such combinations being beneficial. There was one study that compared a stand-alone echinacea supplement with an herbal combination consisting of echinacea, boneset, wild indigo, and arnica. This animal-model study found that the combination product had synergy (that is, it was more powerful as a combination than the constituents were alone) and was more effective at enhancing certain parameters of immune function (Wagner, 1991).

Standardization is the process of ensuring that a particular herb product contains a minimum amount of the active ingredients. However, the active components of echinacea are not definitively known, so standardized products that focus on a particular substance may be neglecting a different substance that could, in future research, prove to be a more important source of health protection. For now, standardized echinacea products are not necessarily preferable.

TIMING IS EVERYTHING

As true for vitamin C and zinc, taking echinacea at the earliest sign of illness has the best chance of waylaying the development of respiratory infections. But if that isn't possible, starting echinacea after the illness has taken hold may still be of benefit to shorten its duration. Remember, divide the total amount of echinacea you plan to take into smaller doses taken every few hours. Keep taking it until your symptoms resolve (up to two weeks).

SAFETY ISSUES AND CONCERNS

Echinacea does not have any known toxic properties. In fact, the only way that one researcher was able to find any sign of harm to the health of cells in a laboratory experiment was ". . . only with very high, clinically irrelevant concentrations" (Coeugniet, 1987). Animals given many times the human therapeutic level of echinacea (in both oral and injection forms) for up to four weeks remained perfectly healthy (Mengs, 1991).

Even though there are no significant side effects from echinacea, there are certain people who should use it cautiously. Since echinacea stimulates the immune system, a concern has been raised that individuals with autoimmune diseases, such as lupus or rheumatoid arthritis, shouldn't take this herb. Though this may make theoretical sense, there is no evidence at this point that echinacea has, over its many years of use, had a negative effect in individuals with such conditions. Nevertheless, we do not recommend the continuous long-term use of echinacea in those with autoimmune conditions until more is known about this issue.

People who have severe allergies to daisies and other flowers in that family (Asteraceae) should only take echinacea under the guidance of a health-care practitioner. There has been one case report of a woman with a history of allergies who had a severe allergic reaction after taking several supplements, including echinacea (Mullins, 1998).

Echinacea in tea or tincture form can make the tongue feel tingly or numb. Don't worry—this is a harmless effect. In fact, as previously mentioned, this tingling sensation is sometimes used to identify products that contain "active" ingredients (although the effectiveness of this informal test is not known).

In the past, many echinacea products on the market were adulterated with another plant: *Parthenium integrifolium L.* (prairie dock). Some of the early research with echinacea has come under scrutiny, since it is not known if the resulting effects were actually based on the echinacea or the prairie dock. Fortunately, this is not the case today; herbal formulas labeled as echinacea are actually true to their labels.

CONCLUSION

Given the importance of starting echinacea at the earliest onset of symptoms, it makes sense to keep a supply of this immune-boosting herb in the house and at the office year-round. This way you'll be ready to start echinacea treatment after your first sneeze, although it will likely offer benefits even if you start it well into the course of illness. Spread your echinacea intake into several smaller doses throughout the day. You can take echinacea in many forms—tea, fluid extract, tincture, or capsules. Echinacea can also be combined with other vitamins, minerals, and herbs.

6 *The Rest of the Herbal Medicine Chest*

Herbs have been the primary source of remedies from time immemorial. Much of the knowledge about the medicinal use of herbs is available today because it was passed down from one generation to the next. Many herbs have been used as tonics, energizers, and immune-system enhancers. Traditional herbal medicine, unlike modern medicine, has paid close attention to the strengthening of the individual's general resistance against infections.

Herbal medicine is sometimes criticized for lacking the hard, scientific research of other types of treatment. Regardless, many years (in some cases, thousands of years) of using herbs safely and effectively should not be discounted just because the modern scientific world is slow to put herbs to the scrutiny of double-blind testing. Having said that, it is hoped that all of the herbs discussed in this chapter will eventually be fully examined by modern standards of research. Please keep in mind that formal research in the medicinal use of herbs is still limited, and until more hard data is available, we have to rely mostly on traditional and anecdotal knowledge, and on the professional experience of herbalists.

This chapter outlines the benefits of a wide number of herbs. For each herb discussed, we cover the traditional and scientific rationale behind its use in the prevention and treatment of respiratory illnesses and their symptoms. We also discuss dosages and necessary precautions. But first, it is important to define the various forms of herbal supplements so that you can become an informed consumer.

FORMS OF HERBAL SUPPLEMENTS

Herbs come in many forms, most of which are effective (except where specifically noted in the text). Basically, this means that you can choose the form that best matches your lifestyle and preferences. For example, we find tinctures and capsules/tablets to be more convenient when we're traveling, but brewing a cup of herbal tea is a soothing, as well as healing, experience when facilities are available. To familiarize you with the lingo of herbal remedies and to help you decide what to purchase, here are some important explanations of the various forms of herbal supplements.

Whole Herbs (Dried or Fresh)

Herbs often come in a minimally processed, whole form, available in bulk at many natural food stores and herb shops. Dried herbs, which are more popular than fresh, should be kept in an airtight container, away from direct sunlight. To use dried herbs, brew them into tea or put them in empty capsules, which are sold in many health food stores and pharmacies.

Teas

Herbal teas are the traditional healing form of herbs. Remember that medicinal herb teas are stronger than the teas that are used simply as beverages and should be taken as directed. To brew herbal tea, place the herb—root, stems, leaves, or whichever is the medicinal part of the herb—in a pot or mug and pour in a cup of boiling water for each teaspoon of herb (unless otherwise directed by the label). Cover and let steep for five to fifteen minutes before drinking. Some herbs are available prepackaged in tea bags.

Many herbal teas have a strong or bitter taste. This can be somewhat masked by sweeteners. We recommend *stevia*, a natural, noncaloric herbal sweetener.

Powdered Herb

Some herbs are sold in powdered form and can be mixed with juice or water. Powdered herbs can also be put into empty capsules, which are sold in pharmacies and health food stores.

Tinctures and Fluid Extracts

There are several ways to extract the active ingredients within herbs. One of the most common is to use alcohol. The resulting concentration is called a tincture. Active ingredients can also be extracted from herbs by simmering the roots, barks, stems, or leaves in boiling water for fifteen to twenty minutes. The result is called a decoction. Decoctions and tinctures are, understandably, much more potent than the tea form.

Capsules/Tablets

Capsules/tablets are perhaps the most common herb forms and get high marks for convenience. Use these supplements as directed by the label; dosages vary greatly according to the herb. Most capsules/tablets are coated with substances that contain gelatin (an animal product). Vegetarians might want to use alternatives, such as veggie "gelatin" or tablets, which are made solely of plant-based materials. The product label should list the ingredients of the coating used. If you have difficulty swallowing capsules or tablets but like the convenience of a pill, check to see if there is a chewable form of the herb you need.

Lozenges

Some herbs are available primarily as lozenges that are designed to be dissolved in the mouth. Slippery elm and licorice are examples of herbs that are best used as lozenges for the relief of a sore throat. Lozenges offer an advantage when it comes to sore throats, as the throat is exposed to the herb's benefits with each swallow.

Herbal Combinations

The combination of two or more herbs in capsules, tablets, extracts, or teas is very common and can be a great way to benefit from herbs that work in concert to support a particular area of health or the relief of symptom(s). Some herbs appear to work better with each other than when taken alone. The increased effectiveness of herbs in combination, as opposed to the effectiveness of each herb taken individually, is referred to as *synergy*. Research with combinations of herbs is extremely limited. If you plan on designing your own combinations, it is best to first consult with an herbalist.

YOUR GUIDE TO HERBS

We have selected a number of herbs to discuss in detail,

because of their convenient availability and their well-known effects in helping to prevent or soothe symptoms of colds and the flu. Some have been researched more extensively than others. Wherever possible, we provide not only traditional uses of the herbs, but information on applicable studies. The dosages and safety precautions that are given are general guidelines. Please consult a health-care professional if you have any concerns or if you take medications that may be affected by the use of herbal remedies.

Astragalus *(Astragalus membranaceus)*

Astragalus has been a popular herb since ancient times among practitioners of Traditional Chinese Medicine. In Chinese medicine, the root of this herb is used as a general tonic, for increased feelings of well-being, as well as for increased resistance to illness. It has recently become popular with American herbalists.

Scientific Background

Laboratory research indicates that compounds within astragalus—substances known as saponins and polysaccharides—stimulate key immune system cells, namely white blood cells (Yoshida, 1997). These white blood cells are then better able to engulf bacteria and other germs. Animal studies have shown that astragalus enhances immune function, especially during times of physical stress (Sugiura, 1993). In addition, a 1995 study conducted in China showed that astragalus was effective in treating patients who had leucopenia, defined as a low white blood cell count (Weng, 1995). After therapy with astragalus, the number of white blood cells of these patients increased significantly.

Some herbalists recommend the combination of astragalus with smaller doses of ginseng to increase immune power in those whose immune systems are weak. Astragalus has been found to promote the release of tumor necrosis factor, a substance that can combat certain cancers (Zhao, 1993).

Usage Recommendations and Cautions

Astragalus is better suited to enhancing immune function in order to prevent illness, rather than to treat an already existing infection. Traditionally, a decoction of astragalus is used. This is made by allowing 5 to 15 grams of the root to boil in water for a few minutes before it is steeped as a tea. This herb is also available in tincture, which can be taken in doses of 3 to 5 milliliters, once or twice per day. Furthermore, it can be taken as a capsule/tablet; take one or two 500-milligram doses, three times daily.

Astragalus, like ginseng, can be used off and on indefinitely. However, during an active cold or flu, it's best to suspend the use of astragalus and other tonic herbs that are taken daily to influence the immune system, since other herbs, such as echinacea, will be substituted. Some herbalists suggest that astragalus should not be used if you have a fever. So it is best not to use this herb if you are actually experiencing a cold or flu.

Astragalus is not currently known to be associated with any side effects. Individuals who wish to use it regularly should take occasional breaks. Long-term effects of chronic use are not fully known.

Boneset *(Eupatorium perfoliatum)*

Several Native American tribes used boneset to treat fevers associated with colds, flu, and other infections, particularly when the infection was associated with muscle and joint aches. The American colonists quickly learned to use this herb in the same manner. However, as aspirin became more popular in the early part of the twentieth century, the use of boneset diminished.

Scientific Background

Despite its popularity in prior centuries, there is a paucity of scientific research on this herb. Preliminary evidence from laboratory experiments indicate that boneset stimulates the function of some aspects of the immune system, particularly by inducing white blood cells to engulf germs (Wagner, 1991).

In a German study, fifty-three outpatients suffering from the common cold or the flu were randomly assigned to either therapy with acetylsalicylic acid (aspirin) or boneset in a controlled clinical trial (Gassinger, 1981). The effectiveness of the therapies was assessed on the first, fourth, and tenth days of the infection. Symptom checklists and physical examinations were the tools of evaluation. The researchers state: "Neither subjective complaints nor body temperature or laboratory findings showed any significant differences between groups. This was taken as evidence that both aspirin and boneset were equally effective."

There is only preliminary scientific evidence that boneset helps treat influenza. Certainly, more studies would shed more light on the effectiveness of this herb as a flu treatment, which was its traditional application.

Usage Recommendations and Cautions

Tea is the traditional medicinal form of boneset. When making boneset tea, use 1 to 2 teaspoons of the herb. Unfortunately, it has a very bitter taste. For this reason, the tincture form is more palatable. If using the boneset tincture, take 2 to 3 milliliters, three times per day.

High doses of boneset, especially the fresh form, can cause nausea and vomiting in some people. Individuals with liver disease should not use this herb. It is also not appropriate for long-term use. To avoid any risk of side effects, use it only for short periods of time during the flu.

Echinacea *(Echinacea purpurea, Echinacea angustifolia, Echinacea pallida)*

Please see Chapter 5 for a detailed description of the history and use of this herb in treating a cold or flu.

Elderberry *(Sambucus nigra)*

Elderberry, also known as black elder, has been a popular food ingredient for many centuries—especially in elderberry pie, wine, and jam. This plant grows in both Europe and North America and has a lengthy history. In Roman times, elderberry was considered a flu remedy, which remains its forté even today. In Europe, juice and cordials made from the elderberry herb were used for colds—especially chest colds—and as a spring tonic. Elderberry tea was also recommended by herbalists for colds and sore throats. The primary uses of elderberry cited by Native Americans long ago were for coughs, infections, and skin conditions.

Scientific Background

Elderberry extract was studied for its ability to treat influenza in Israel, during an outbreak at a kibbutz or collective farm (Zakay-Rones, 1995). The double-blind, clinical trial provided either elderberry extract or a placebo to twenty-seven adults and children who had contracted the flu. The study participants suffered from typical flu symptoms—namely fever, muscle aches, nasal discharge, and cough—for less than twenty-four hours before the study began. For three days, half of the participants took the elderberry and the other half took the placebos. Their symptoms were tracked for a total of six days.

Within the first twenty-four hours of starting the study, 20 percent of the individuals in the elderberry group reported that their symptoms of fever, cough, and muscle pain significantly improved. After another day, 75 percent were greatly improved, while by the third day, 90 percent of the elderberry users reported a complete cure. In comparison, 8 percent of the control group improved in the first day, but it took until the sixth day for 92 percent of these individuals to recover.

The elderberry-treated group had higher levels of antibodies than the placebo group, indicating that the elderberry stimulated immune response. The research team also reported that in laboratory experiments, elderberry extract has an antiviral effect by preventing the influenza virus from entering the cell—which means that the virus can't easily replicate itself to cause an infection.

Usage Recommendations and Cautions

Elderberry is best reserved for use during a flu attack, rather than used for daily maintenance throughout the year. It seems to work most effectively when its use is started within twenty-four hours of the first symptom. Elderberry tea is the traditional way this herb was given to treat colds, the flu, and sore throats. Several cups of elderberry tea can be drunk each day. It has the added benefit of replenishing fluids to a flu-battered body.

The standardized liquid extract of elderberry is the form used successfully in research for the treatment of the flu. If you are using the liquid extract form, the recommended dosage is 5 milliliters for children, and 10 milliliters for adults, taken twice per day. If you are using the tablet/capsule form, take 100 to 200 milligrams, three to four times daily. If treating a child with elderberry, use one-half or one-third of the adult dose. Be sure to read and follow label directions.

The *Sambucus nigra* species of elderberry is not known to have any side effects. However, there are other species of elderberry that are toxic. For this reason, care should be taken that black elder (*Sambucus nigra*) is the species used.

Ephedra *(Ephedra sinica)*

See Ma Huang.

Garlic *(Allium sativum)*

Garlic has been called the "poor person's antibiotic," indicating this herb's role in treating various infections. Garlic, as well as the related herbs onions and chives, have been used therapeutically throughout human history, not only for the prevention and treatment of infections, but also for digestive complaints, circulatory health, and as overall tonics.

Scientific Background

Garlic has been the topic of numerous studies on enhanced immune function, although many of these studies are based on laboratory experiments rather than clinical trials. Such laboratory studies show that garlic increases resistance to disease by stimulating the activity of lymphocytes, which are a type of white blood cell, and increasing the production of phagocytes, which are cells that engulf and digest foreign invaders (Lau, 1990). Studies in humans have found that garlic stimulates immunity by increasing the number of natural killer cells, as well as improving the function of other parts of the immune system (Hughes, 1991).

Usage Recommendation and Cautions

Garlic is better suited as a preventive, rather than a treatment, of colds and the flu. As such, incorporating a clove or more of garlic into your daily diet is a tasty way to benefit from this herb. Supplements of garlic are also an option. The tincture should be taken in doses of 2 to 4 milliliters, three times per day. Capsules/tablets come in odor-controlled forms and are safe for daily supplementation, if you choose.

Garlic intake is generally harmless, although some people develop heartburn and/or flatulence. This herb has a slight blood-thinning effect, which is beneficial for many people, but individuals who are using anticoagulant drugs or who are about to have surgery should inform their health-care providers.

Ginger *(Zingiber officinale)*

Ginger has been a widely revered healer around the world. It is a common therapeutic herb, particularly in Traditional Chinese Medicine, which has used it for 2,500 years, as well as in India and the West Indies. The main health benefits traditionally attributed to ginger are relief from abdominal upset, vomiting, diarrhea, rheumatism, and coughing. A survey of Indian mothers reports that ginger, usually made as a warm tea with honey, remains a popular home remedy for treating childhood respiratory infections—especially coughs—even in modern times (Mishra, 1994).

Scientific Background

Most of the research with ginger centers around nausea associated with motion sickness, pregnancy, and post-surgical illness. However, there are a small number of studies that support the traditional use of ginger for symptom relief during a cold. An animal study found that an extract of ginger root reduced fever and had an antibacterial effect (Mascolo, 1989). Furthermore, a laboratory experiment demonstrated ginger to have a direct effect on inhibiting the rhinovirus—the virus responsible for about half of all colds (Denyer, 1994).

Usage Recommendations and Cautions

Ginger's underground stem, called the rhizome, is the medicinal part of the herb. It is available in quite a few forms, including powder, tea, tincture, capsules/tablets, and even the whole herb used in cooking. If you like ginger tea, which is often made with honey and lemon, you may drink up to several cups per day. Alternately, 2 to 3 milliliters of a ginger tincture, taken three times daily, or a total of 1 gram of ginger taken in capsule/tablet form, can be used. This herb may help ease nausea in patients with the flu. No side effects of any significance have been reported with its use.

Ginseng *(Eleutherococcus senticosus, Panax ginseng)*

Ginseng has been in traditional use by Chinese medicine for thousands of years, namely as a general tonic and to boost vitality in the elderly. Asian ginseng (*Panax ginseng*, also called Korean ginseng or Chinese ginseng) was usually applied in this energizing role. Siberian ginseng (*Eleutherococcus senticosus,* or eleuthero) is a distant relative to Asian ginseng and was recommended in Chinese medicine for colds and flu prevention, as well as for energy support.

Scientific Background

The research on the immune-boosting (cold-fighting) ability of the various ginsengs is limited. However, there is a double-blind study that examined the effect of a standardized ginseng extract during influenza vaccination (Scaglione, 1996). A standardized extract contains certain levels of active ingredients of the herb. This study, which included 227 adults, provided either daily placebos or daily ginseng supplements containing 100 milligrams of standardized extract. The study lasted for twelve weeks. During the fourth week of supplementation, everyone was given a vaccination against influenza. From the time of the vaccination until the end of the study, the incidence of colds and flu was tracked. There were forty-two cases in the placebo group, but only fifteen cases in the ginseng group, indicating that the ginseng induced a higher immune response after vaccination against influenza.

Usage Recommendations and Cautions

Ginseng's role is more of an immune-system stimulant to prevent infections rather than an herb to treat an infection once it has occurred. Small doses of ginseng can be used on a regular basis. However, ginseng, similarly to astragalus, should not be used continuously; for every month of use, take a break of a week or two.

Ginseng is available in a panoply of forms, including tea, capsules/tablets, and tincture. In capsule/tablet form, take 100 to 200 milligrams per day of the standardized extract, or 500 milligrams of the root powder. In tincture form, take 5 to 10 milliliters per day. Ginseng can be combined with small doses of astragalus for immune enhancement. Please keep in mind that countless dosages and products of ginseng are sold. As a rule, follow the instructions on the label of the specific product you choose. And if you are sensitive to stimulants, take a lesser amount.

Due to its energizing effects, ginseng can cause insomnia in some people, especially when taken later in the day. During an active cold or flu, it's best to suspend the use of ginseng and other tonic herbs that are taken daily to influence the immune system, since other herbs, such as echinacea, should be substituted for better help in treating the illness.

Goldenseal (Hydrastis canadensis)

Goldenseal is a Native American herb. It was traditionally used to fight infections, including upper respiratory tract infections, as well as to relieve irritations of the digestive tract, the skin, and the eyes. Native Americans introduced American colonists to this herb, and the colonists incorporated it into their treatment therapies for many of the same purposes. Goldenseal remains popular today as a cold-fighter, although the scientific research in this regard is lacking.

Scientific Background

Most of the research involving goldenseal is limited in scope to one of goldenseal's ingredients—berberine—although goldenseal has other potentially active constituents. Berberine is also found in other herbs, including barberry, Oregon grape root, gold thread, and Yerba mansa. This substance has been shown to have an antibacterial effect against many species of bacteria (Hahn, 1976).

It should be noted that there is no solid documentation that goldenseal or other berberine-containing herbs will aid in the prevention or recovery of colds and the flu, particularly since these conditions are caused by viruses, and most of the berberine research is related to bacteria. However, there is some evidence that berberine stimulates the activity of some immune system cells (Kumazawa, 1984). This stimulation may be applicable to cold and flu therapies.

Usage Recommendations and Cautions

Goldenseal is sometimes used in combination with other herbs, especially echinacea. Tea can be made from goldenseal root (or the other berberine-containing herbs). Berberine is not easily soluble in water, though, so capsules/tablets or liquid extracts (often standardized for berberine content) may be a better choice. A goldenseal tincture is also available. Dosages are highly dependent upon the specific product you select. Therefore, follow label directions for the supplementation of goldenseal and other berberine-containing herbs.

Although there are no strong concerns about gold-enseal (or other berberine-containing herbs), high intakes of berberine can cause stomach upset and, possibly, nervous system effects, especially when the stronger standardized extracts are used. These herbs are best not used by pregnant or lactating women.

Due to the popularity of goldenseal, it is necessary to include a discussion of its role in cold and flu treatment. However, at this time, we do not recommend the use of goldenseal in the prevention or therapy of colds and the flu. It's possible that future research will indicate that this herb plays a role in fighting these viral infections. But for the time being, based on the available evidence, we prefer that you rely on some of the other herbs that we recommend throughout this book.

Green Tea *(Camellia sinensis)*

Green tea has been used in Traditional Chinese Medicine for a wide variety of applications, including as a general tonic and to promote digestion, stimulate mental clarity, boost immunity, energize the body, and prolong life. It is now popular in American health markets.

Scientific Background

The active constituents of green tea (as well as black tea and oolong tea) are substances called polyphenols. Polyphenols enhance immune function and also have a direct effect to minimize the infectiousness of certain germs. According to animal model studies, polyphenols boost lymphocyte activity (Hu, 1992). These polyphenols—namely EGCG, or epigallocatechin gallate—interfere with the ability of viruses to attach to cells, and thereby have an antiviral effect (Mukoyama, 1991).

Research relating to green tea and the flu is more prolific than that related to the common cold. Laboratory research conducted with the influenza virus suggests that EGCG binds with this virus to prevent infections (Nakayama, 1993). Animal research has found similar results (Nakayama, 1994).

Usage Recommendations and Cautions

About one or two cups of green tea can be drunk most days, to provide a mild immune boost and possibly lessen the risk of infection during the cold and flu season. If you prefer pill forms, capsules/tablets containing standardized amounts of polyphenols are available. Suggested daily intake is about 250 to 750 milligrams of green tea daily.

Green tea does contain small amounts of caffeine. If the tea is taken in large amounts, sensitive individuals may experience insomnia or anxiety. As an alternative, there are decaffeinated green tea extracts available.

On a side note, black tea also appears to have benefits. In one study, adults who gargled with black tea twice daily were less likely to catch the flu—even when they were exposed to the virus—compared with adults who didn't gargle with black tea (Iwata, 1997).

Licorice *(Glycyrrhiza glabra)*

Licorice has been used since ancient times as a flavoring, as well as for medicinal purposes during a cold to soothe coughs and help expel mucus. It is found in Europe and Asia. Herbalists also note that licorice has demulcent, or throat-soothing, properties. Don't confuse the herb with the artificial flavoring. Today, most "licorice" candy is flavored with anise.

Scientific Background

There is laboratory evidence that licorice has a general antimicrobial effect (Okada, 1989). And animal research shows that a constituent of licorice called *glycyrrhizin* has antiviral activity, specifically against the influenza virus (Utsunomiya, 1997).

Usage Recommendations and Cautions

A few cups of tea made from licorice root can be drunk during a cold or flu to help quell a cough, encourage the expulsion of mucus, and generally aid in healing. Similarly, licorice lozenges (or even licorice candies, if they are made with real licorice) can be taken for these purposes.

If using capsules/tablets or tincture of licorice, take care that the products are not "deglycyrrhizated licorice," often seen as "DGL." These products do not contain the glycyrrhizin substance that has been shown to have antiviral properties. The reason that some licorice preparations are formulated as deglycyrrhizated is because the glycyrrhizin component of licorice can increase blood pressure and lead to water retention. For adequate capsule/tablet supplementation, take 3 to 6 grams per day. For adequate tincture supplementation, take 2 to 5 milliliters, one to three times per day.

Short-term (that is, a few days) use of licorice with glycyrrhizin is fine for most people, with the exception of anyone who has high blood pressure. Such individuals might consider other herbs discussed in this chapter in place of licorice. Licorice should not be used for prolonged periods by anyone, unless under the supervision of a physician.

Ma Huang (*Ephedra sinica*)

Ma huang, also known as ephedra, is an herb derived from the *Ephedra sinica* plant. It is the first known cultivated medicinal plant. Ma huang has a recorded therapeutic history going back more than 5,000 years in Traditional Chinese Medicine. Traditionally, the primary uses for ma huang were for the alleviation of colds, flu, coughs, nasal congestion, headache, fever, chills, asthma, and hay fever.

Scientific Background

The active ingredients in the ma huang herb are ephedrine and pseudoephedrine. Because of their decongestant effects, both act as central nervous system stimulants, open up constricted bronchial tubes, and relieve nasal congestion. This herb has been put to the test in several studies and is confirmed to be effective in relieving some symptoms of colds. In fact, the Food and Drug Administration has approved the use of ephedrine and pseudoephedrine as active ingredients in over-the-counter remedies for the common cold, flu, and asthma.

Usage Recommendations and Cautions

Ma huang should be used cautiously and in small amounts for the relief of symptoms during an upper respiratory tract infection. Follow label directions for teas and tinctures. If capsules/tablets containing ephedrine are used, adults should limit daily intake to a maximum of 10 milligrams per dose, with a maximum of 30 milligrams daily.

Ma huang is generally safe in small amounts for short-term use. However, large amounts of this herb (and especially ephedrine extracted from the herb) have been used inappropriately for weight loss and for energy boosting. There have been reports of heart palpitations, nervousness, and even death from heart failure in those with extremely high intakes of ma huang. In addition, certain individuals should avoid ma huang altogether, including the following: those who are pregnant or lactating; those who have high blood pressure, heart or thyroid disease, diabetes, or enlarged prostate; and those who use MAO inhibiting drugs, which are taken for the treatment of depression.

Marshmallow *(Althea officinalis)*

European herbalists have primarily used marshmallow for easing coughs and sore throats. (The herb marshmallow should not be confused with the fluffy candy that is similar in name only.) The roots and leaves of the marshmallow plant contain a substance called *mucilage,* which soothes the lining of the throat, as well as other parts of the digestive tract.

Scientific Background

There is scant research on this herb. However, although anecdotal, the soothing qualities of its mucilage are generally not disputed for coughs and sore throats.

Usage Recommendations and Cautions

For the symptoms of cough or sore throat, marshmallow made into a tea is the preferable form. However, the herbalist Janet Zand reports that in her herbal practice, she has found that gargling with marshmallow or using a marshmallow throat spray is also effective. The tincture and capsule/tablet forms are not recommended for coughs and sore throat, since they do not act directly on the throat. Side effects, with the exception of a very rare allergic reaction, are not seen with marshmallow use.

Meadowsweet *(Filipendula ulmaria)*

See White Willow.

Mullein *(Verbascum thapsus)*

The leaves and flowers of the mullein plant are best known by European herbalists for their expectorant and demulcent properties. This means that mullein helps break up and expel mucus, while soothing a sore throat. Mullein is recognized for its mucilage content (see page 91), and is generally available in the United States.

Scientific Background

As with marshmallow, the mucilage in mullein accounts for the soothing qualities that this herb provides for the throat. However, other constituents may account for the expectorant activity. There are no studies concerning mullein, but many herbalists confirm that it is effective.

Usage Recommendations and Cautions

Mullein is used primarily to ease the sore throat associated with upper respiratory tract infections. Tea made from the dried leaves or flowers of the mullein plant is probably the best form of this herb, since warm liquids have other benefits for a sore throat, as well. It is helpful to strain the tea to remove the hairs, which can be irritating. A tincture form is also available; take 1 to 4 milliliters, several times daily. Mullein is not known to be associated with any side effects.

Mushrooms *(Maitake, Reishi, Shiitake)*

Several species of mushrooms have long been utilized medicinally in Asia, particularly maitake, reishi, and shiitake. They have been used historically as general tonics, to promote overall wellness and vitality. Some traditional herbalists also recommend these mushrooms for the treatment of colds and coughs.

Scientific Background

Modern scientific research has focused on the complex polysaccharides (sugar-based molecules) in maitake, reishi, and shiitake. Research has shown that these components enhance the immune system in its fight against cancer prevention and in AIDS treatment (Chang, 1996). There is a clear immune function benefit from the consumption of these mushrooms, but there is a lack of scientific documentation for the role of maitake, reishi, or shiitake in the prevention or treatment of colds and the flu. Even so, many herbalists recommend the use of medicinal mushrooms for general immune enhancement during the cold and flu season.

Usage Recommendations and Cautions

Consuming the whole, dried mushrooms is the traditional way to use maitake, reishi, and shiitake. However, other forms can sometimes be more convenient, including tinctures, capsules/tablets, and powder. In tincture form, take 2 to 4 milliliters per day; the same tincture dose generally applies for each type of mushroom. In capsule/tablet and powder forms, take 2 to 6 grams daily of maitake, 1 to 1.5 grams daily of reishi, and 5 to 15 grams daily of shiitake. You can also get teas made from these mushrooms.

The use of mushrooms is a preventive step, as opposed to acute therapy. As with the other herbs, such as astragulas and ginseng, take breaks when using mushrooms over the long term. During an active cold or flu attack, it's best to suspend the use of mushrooms that are taken daily to influence the immune system, as other herbs, such as echinacea, will be used in substitution.

Maitake is not associated with any side effects. Reishi can cause symptoms such as dizziness, dry mouth, and upset stomach. Shiitake has been reported to cause temporary diarrhea at high doses.

Slippery Elm (*Ulmus rubra*)

Native American healers utilized slippery elm internally for sore throats and diarrhea, and externally for many skin ailments. Slippery elm's inner bark, much like marshmallow and mullein, contains mucilage, a substance that is generally effective for soothing a sore throat.

Scientific Background

Unfortunately, there is only traditional use to back this herb. Hopefully, studies will be conducted in the future, as slippery elm has long been recognized to be helpful for sore throats.

Usage Recommendations and Cautions

Forms of slippery elm that put this herb into contact with a sore throat—that is, lozenges, syrups and tinctures (5 milliliters, three times daily), and tea—provide temporary symptom relief. Capsules/tablets do not provide relief from cold symptoms, as they don't allow direct action on the throat. Janet Zand, an experienced herbalist, reports that slippery elm is very effective in easing sore throat, and that gargling with tea or syrup is a good option. And slippery elm lozenges are a permanent part of Mrs. Toews' cold/flu season medicine kit. She has found relief from many episodes of sore throat with this herb. Furthermore, there are no known side effects associated with the use of this herb. It can be used as needed to relieve a sore throat.

White Willow (*Salix alba*)

Bark from the white willow tree is an herbal source of salicin, a compound similar to aspirin. Other herbs also contain this aspirin-like compound, including meadowsweet. Salicin was used traditionally for pain relief, to lower fever, to ease headaches, and to provide relief from arthritic conditions. (Aspirin is much more potent.) It is native to Europe and North America, where it has been used as a traditional medicine.

Scientific Background

White willow is used on the basis of knowledge established by herbalists. Studies done on this herb date too far back to be applicable to today's standards.

Usage Recommendations and Cautions

White willow can be taken in tincture, capsule/tablet, or tea form, whichever you prefer. The tincture should be taken in doses of 1 to 2 milliliters, three times per day. In capsule/tablet form, a daily total of 60 to 120 milligrams of salicin is effective. The effects of the tea will be much weaker than the tincture or capsules/tablets. And in any form, don't expect white willow to be as powerful as aspirin.

Individuals who are allergic to aspirin should not take white willow, just in case they are also allergic to salicin, nor should children younger than age fourteen. Also, continual use of white willow for prolonged periods of time could result in stomach upset or ulcers. As with aspirin, white willow should not be given to children because of the theoretical risk of Reye's syndrome, a neurological condition that could be fatal. However, a connection between white willow and Reye's syndrome has not been reported in medical literature.

Meadowsweet is another herb that contains salicin and probably additional anti-clotting agents. It can be substituted for white willow. The same cautions apply.

Wild Cherry *(Prunus serotina)*

The bark of the wild cherry tree has a long history of use by Native Americans for treating coughs. And wild cherry syrup has been used traditionally to ease coughs by many herbalists. It is very commonly found in cold preparations.

Scientific Background

It is thought that substances in the wild cherry plant can reduce spasms in the lungs and therefore ease coughing fits. Adequate research is not yet available to determine whether wild cherry works mostly as an antitussive—a substance that reduces the cough reflex—or mostly as an expectorant, loosening mucus.

Usage Recommendations and Cautions

Either the syrup or the tincture of wild cherry can be used to ease the symptoms of a cough. Take 1 teaspoon of either, several times daily. In exceptionally large amounts for prolonged periods, wild cherry could theoretically produce cyanide toxicity, as cyanide is potentially one of its components. However, there is no clinical evidence of this happening. Wild cherry is safe to use in small amounts for the short-term relief of a cough related to a cold.

A WORD OF CAUTION

Herbal remedies are generally safe when used as directed. However, certain combinations of herbs and over-the-counter or prescription drugs can have undesirable interactions. For instance, ma huang can interact negatively when used in combination with certain antidepressants. For this reason, if you are using any medications, it is a good idea to inform your physician about which herbs you are taking.

CONCLUSION

This chapter touched on herbal highlights when it comes to strengthening the immune function and easing the many symptoms associated with respiratory tract infections. From the information in this chapter, it is evident that there are many natural ways to address the undesirable symptoms of upper respiratory infections this cold and flu season. As modern researchers examine the healing potential of plants more closely, more herbs are bound to be recognized and validated as supportive during the cold and flu season. It is also possible that research will find that certain traditional recommendations are not supported by double-blind studies. Regardless of what studies have and have not been done as of yet, we cannot disregard the valuable wealth of traditional and anecdotal knowledge to which we have access from various ancient systems of medicine. In the following chapter, you'll find out how to put herbs, vitamins, and other natural remedies into action to prevent, cure, or treat cold and flu symptoms.

7

Practical Ways to Conquer a Cold and Fight a Flu

E ach year, the average American suffers through several uncomfortable episodes of sniffles and sneezes—but your name doesn't have to be on this casualty list. By going on the nutritional offensive, choosing the appropriate supplements, and maintaining healthy habits, you can keep yourself free of winter misery. This chapter gives you specific dietary and lifestyle tips on how to fight off common cold and flu viruses. It also offers you day-by-day, step-by-step plans to get rid of an infection if one has caught you off guard.

YOUR PLAN FOR A BETTER IMMUNE DEFENSE

Developing a strong, resilient immune system is your best protection against germ invaders. Immune function is very complex and influenced by a number of factors. Just about every dietary and lifestyle choice you make will, in either a minor or a significant way, affect the effectiveness of your immune defense. The bottom line is that it's not so much which germ you are exposed to, but how well your immune system can block its entry and thwart its advances that determines your health status. And building up a strong immune system long before you are exposed to the latest bug visiting your community is your best option for giving the next cold virus the cold shoulder. Chapter 1 discussed general enhancement of the immune system. Here's more information that we'd really like to emphasize so that you can do the best job of avoiding that cold or flu.

Consume a Proper Diet

Dietary advice is grouped into two areas: foods you should emphasize in your diet, and those you should limit or avoid, in order to strengthen your immune defense.

Foods to Put on Your Plate. Immune-enhancing foods tend to be those that are the least processed and the closest to their whole, unadulterated state. Fruits, vegetables, whole-grain breads and cereals, and beans and legumes are the power foods in this area. Of these, fruits and vegetables are particularly important because they are the richest food sources of vitamins, as well as phytonutrients such as carotenoids and flavonoids. Phytonutrients are naturally occurring substances found in many plants that promote health and fight disease. For example, many phytonutrients have antiviral properties. Aim for at least five servings of fruits and vegetables every day.

Yogurt and other fermented foods also contribute to healthy immune function. They provide beneficial bacteria. Garlic and onions enhance immunity too, as explained on pages 82 to 83. All of these are great additions to the daily diet.

Let's not forget the good fats. Essential fatty acids, especially the omega-3 fatty acids, are important for proper immune function. They are found in cold-water fish and some vegetable oils. Because of their fat profile, canola and flaxseed oil are preferable choices to safflower, sunflower, or corn oil. The former contain omega-3s. Olive oil is not an omega-3 oil, but is a healthy choice. See the "Healthy Eating Habits" section of Chapter 1 (beginning on page 15) for more information on good diet.

Foods to Keep Off Your Plate. The foods that should be limited or avoided in your diet shouldn't come as a surprise—they're the foods your mother frequently warned you against overindulging. Limit your intake of refined carbohydrates (sugars), since sugar hinders the germ-fighting ability of the immune system (Ringsdorf, 1976). Sugar is often plentiful in sodas, cereal, baked goods, and other processed foods. A diet high in fats—especially the trans-fats found in fried foods, margarine, and baked goods—interferes with the ability of certain immune cells to destroy invaders (Kubena, 1996).

Also, avoid alcohol binges. Excessive alcohol intake dampens immune function (Ahmed, 1995). Moderate consumption of alcohol is not known to interfere with immune function (Cohen, 1993).

Run, Relax, and Relate for Health

Regular physical activity is a crucial component of optimum health, vigor, and long-term maintenance of a healthy immune system. Studies show that exercise boosts the activity of natural killer cells—white blood cells that have a talent for seeking out and destroying viruses (Nieman, 1994). Regular exercise will help keep your organs healthy and will allow you to sleep better.

Quality rest is essential for maintaining health. Most people do well with six to eight hours of deep sleep every night. Sleep interruption is known to decrease the number and effectiveness of natural killer cells. Hence, inadequate sleep, even in the short run, can make you more suscepti-ble to viruses.

There is no doubt that stress, whether physical, emo-tional, or mental, is a powerful immune drainer. The per-ception of stress by the brain leads to the release of stress hormones, which travel to the adrenal glands and increase the release of cortisol. Cortisol is a hormone known to se-verely depress almost all aspects of the immune system. Individuals who are treated with cortisol or related medi-cines for specific medical conditions, such as lupus, some-times come down with severe infections.

The physical stress of intense exercise or even a pre-existing illness or infection can make you more vulnerable to catching a cold. Emotional or mental stressors can have a similar effect. Incorporating stress management into your daily life is a great way to feel better while benefiting your immune system. Some suggestions are yoga, tai chi, medi-tation, prayer, and keeping a journal.

Conversely, positive emotions and satisfying social relationships have an uplifting effect on immunity. When 276 volunteers were exposed to one of the viruses that cause the common cold, those most socially involved—those who were working, involved in family activites, involved in sports, church, etc.—were four times less like-ly to actually succumb to the cold virus (Cohen, 1997). So ultimately, having social involvement, emotional support, and being involved in diverse activities provides some protection from the cold virus. Still, it's not all bad news for singles. The risk of exposure to cold germs is signifi-cantly diminished for those living alone.

Boost Immunity with Vitamin and Mineral Supplements

Almost every single vitamin and mineral biochemically contributes to proper immune function, but there are a few standouts that you might want to consider incorporating into your nutritional supplement regimen to bolster your resistance to infections. For a general list of recommendations, see the "Important Immune-Boosting Supplements" section of Chapter 1 (pages 17 to 18). More details on the ones we find especially applicable to cold and flu prevention and treatment are offered below.

Multivitamin/mineral. A well-balanced multivitamin/ mineral providing most of the essential vitamins and minerals is a great starting place to provide your immune system with required building blocks. Make sure adequate amounts of the B vitamins (especially vitamin B_6, folic acid, and vitamin B_{12}) are included in the supplement.

Multivitamins/minerals act as broad-spectrum insurance, complementing a healthy diet to ensure that basic nutritional needs are met. A daily multiple is particularly important for the many people who have nutritional gaps in their diets, often due to weight-loss diets, eating on the run, or relying on processed or empty-calorie foods.

Think about your lifestyle when choosing a multivitamin/mineral. The once-daily type makes sense for people who have trouble remembering or are too busy to take several pills each day. On the other hand, multiples that are designed to be taken in several smaller dosages throughout the day provide nutrients more evenly and allow flexibility to take more or fewer pills.

When choosing a multiple, take the time to do a little comparison shopping. For basic nutritional insurance, a supplement supplying about 100 to 300 percent of the Recommended Dietary Allowances (RDAs) for most of the B vitamins, and 50 to 100 percent for most of the minerals, is a good place to start. The RDAs are the baseline recommended amounts of nutrients required by healthy people.

Regardless of which multivitamin/mineral supplement is chosen, it's best to take it with a meal, since nausea is less likely to occur when you don't have an empty stomach. Whatever supplement you choose, take care to store it in a cool, dark place, since heat and light can degrade some of the nutrients over time. Importantly, many of the nutrients suggested for supplementation in the following paragraphs are present in adequate amounts in multivitamin/mineral supplements and an extra supplement may not be necessary or beneficial.

Omega-3 Fatty Acids (Fish Oil). If you don't normally include fish in your diet, consider supplementing daily with fish oil capsules. Omega-3s help the immune cells to work better. A dose of 500 to 1,000 milligrams of a combination of EPA and DHA (the active constituents of fish oil) is adequate. Other sources of omega-3 fatty acids include flaxseed oil and (in lesser amounts) canola oil.

Vitamin A. Vitamin A is crucial for a well-running immune system. Deficiencies of this vitamin put the odds in favor of the microorganisms, allowing easier penetration of mucous membranes (Glaszious, 1993). Conversely, adequate intake of this vitamin reduces the risk of infection (West, 1991). Individuals can take 5,000 to 10,000 international units (IU) of this vitamin daily. More likely than not, your multivitamin will already include this amount of vitamin A.

It is generally not recommended that you take larger amounts, since vitamin A can accumulate in your body. Long-term use of very high amounts, such as 30,000 international units daily or greater, can cause toxicity. Women of child-bearing age should be particularly careful to limit vitamin A intake to no more than 10,000 international units daily, since higher amounts are linked to an increased risk of birth defects. Beta-carotene is a precursor to vitamin A and can be used more safely at a wider range of intakes.

Vitamin C. As Chapter 3 explains in detail, vitamin C is a very important nutrient for maintaining optimal immunity

Top Ten Tips for Ducking a Cold

It's a germy world out there, but there are some steps you and your family can take to protect yourself from being infected with the latest virus circulating around your home or office:

- Wash your hands frequently, and avoid shaking hands with someone who has a cold.

- Keep your hands away from your eyes and nose. Most colds are transmitted to the respiratory system when we touch our faces.

- Maintain moist mucous membranes, which physically block the entrance of viral invaders, by drinking plenty of water, wearing lip balm, and using a humidifier during the cold, dry season.

- Use a facial tissue when sneezing or coughing.

- Get deep sleep—at least six to eight hours a night.

- Eat plenty of fruits, vegetables, and whole foods.

- Limit your intake of alcohol, caffeine, and sugar.

- Incorporate immune-boosting supplements.

- Be physically active.

- Take the time to laugh, relax, and enjoy social interactions.

and reducing the severity and duration of the common cold. For year-round immune enhancement, supplement with 100 to 250 milligrams of vitamin C once or twice per day. If cold or flu symptoms start to emerge, take 3 to 5 grams immediately, and then another gram every two to three hours thereafter. Reduce your intake if you experience gastrointestinal upset.

Vitamin E. Infections caused by viruses are known to deplete the body of antioxidant nutrients. Antioxidants protect the body from free radicals—harmful molecules that damage body tissues—and play an important role in optimal immune function. Vitamin E, in particular, has demonstrated its effectiveness in strengthening immunity and infection resistance. The effect of vitamin E is especially important in the elderly. Studies focused on influenza show, in animal models, that the flu lowers vitamin E levels in the body (Hennet, 1992); but when mice are given high doses of vitamin E, this vitamin bolsters resistance to the flu in older animals. Younger animals who have not yet experienced the age-related decline in immune function gained only a slight benefit from vitamin E for influenza resistance (Hayek, 1997).

A daily vitamin E intake of 30 to 200 international units per day is adequate. Choose the natural form of vitamin E, which is listed on the label as d-alpha-tocopherol or RRR-alpha-tocopherol, as opposed to the synthetic form, which is listed on the label as dl-alpha tocopherol or all-rac-alpha-tocopherol (Burton, 1998). An even better option is taking a supplement that includes the full spectrum of natural vitamin E. Supplements of this type are often labeled as vitamin E complex and are readily available in stores.

Selenium. Selenium stimulates the function of certain immune system cells, while a deficiency of this mineral increases the risk of infection. Natural selenium, found under the name selenium-rich yeast or L-selenomethionine, is more easily utilized by the body than other forms of selenium. This mineral can be taken in the approximate amount of 50 micrograms. It's quite likely that your multivitamin/mineral will contain this amount of selenium.

Zinc. As Chapter 4 discusses, the mineral zinc improves immune function in deficient individuals. A daily intake of 5 to 15 milligrams is advised, but will most likely be found in your multivitamin/mineral. Zinc lozenges, however, are best suited for when a cold or flu actually hits, as opposed to supplemental use for prevention, and we highly recommend them. Please see pages 56 to 57 for cautionary information regarding zinc supplementation.

Help Your Health With Herbs

Garlic and onions contain several components that inhibit the growth of microorganisms and stimulate the immune system. If you do not incorporate these pungent herbs in your diet, consider garlic supplements. Also, echinacea (see Chapter 5) is effective when used at the very start of a cold, to nip the infection in the bud. Astragalus and ginseng are other immune-stimulating herbs that can be taken in small dosages off-and-on throughout the year. Refer to Chapter 6 for details on these and other herbs, and Chapter 8 for suggestions for specific symptoms.

So through healthy foods, exercise, rest, social activity, good supplementation, and several potent herbs, you can truly do a good job of preventing the common cold and the flu. But just in case you catch one, we're going to help you get through it as quickly and comfortably as possible.

YOUR PLAN OF ATTACK IF A COLD VIRUS INVADES

Your best efforts at creating a germ-proof immune system have failed. What now? This section explains—hour by hour, day by day—how to stop a cold before it settles in for a lengthy stay.

This supplement plan has the best chances of being effective the earlier you start. So pay close attention to your body, and start supplementing at the first moment that you suspect a cold is coming on. Cold symptoms usually develop about two or three days after you are exposed to a germ. It helps to keep your home stocked with the most crucial supplements year-round, so that you can achieve the fastest response time.

IMMEDIATE ACTIONS

When you notice the first symptom of a cold—often a scratchy throat, runny nose, a tingling sensation in your nose or throat, or sneezing, take the following steps:

- Take 3 to 5 grams of vitamin C. You may wish to stock 500-milligram tablets/capsules and take six to ten of these.

- Allow a zinc lozenge containing 10 to 23 milligrams of zinc in the form of zinc gluconate, zinc gluconate/glycine, or zinc acetate to dissolve in your mouth. It doesn't hurt to use a zinc lozenge right away, even if you're not sure that your vague symptoms will result in a cold. Keep this lozenge in your mouth for as long as you can—for a minimum of five to ten minutes. Swallowing the lozenge early will reduce the time necessary for the zinc to be absorbed into the tissues of the mouth and throat.

- Echinacea can be used in whichever form you prefer: tea made from 1 gram of the herb for every cup of boiling water; 3 to 5 milliliters (5 milliliters equals one teaspoon) of alcohol-, water-, or glycerin-based fluid extract; 3 to 5 milliliters tincture; or 200 to 400 milligrams in capsules/tablets.

- Drink extra fluids. Water and herbal teas, such as peppermint, ginger, and chamomile, are great choices.

THE FIRST DAY

When it comes to fighting a cold, the first couple of hours are crucial. Every two to three hours for the rest of the first day of treatment, follow these guidelines for continued help:

- Take 1 gram of vitamin C.

- Dissolve one zinc lozenge in your mouth. If symptoms are not improved, you can use zinc up to every hour. One drawback to this frequent use is palate irritation.

- Echinacea can be used in whichever form you prefer; see the guidelines on page 108.

THE FIRST NIGHT

If your symptoms have persisted to bedtime, we recommend using the therapy listed under "The First Day" immediately before you retire for the night. And if you wake up in the middle of the night, at least allow a zinc lozenge to melt in your mouth for a few minutes. In our experience, we have found that even when symptoms are controlled the first day, the symptoms are likely to return by morning if the virus is given a breather overnight.

THE SECOND DAY

During the second day of symptoms, continue drinking extra fluids throughout the day. Rest if you feel fatigued, and use a humidifier if your nasal passages feel dry. Every three to four hours, do the following:

- Take 500 milligrams of vitamin C.

- Dissolve one zinc lozenge in your mouth. Actually, if you can tolerate it, it's best to take a zinc lozenge every two to three hours.

• Echinacea can be used in whichever form you prefer; see the guidelines on page 108.

THE FOLLOWING DAYS

Continue drinking extra fluids, resting, and using a humidifier in your bedroom. Finally, this advice should be followed until your symptoms are resolved:

• Take 500 milligrams of vitamin C twice a day.

• Dissolve one zinc lozenge in your mouth every few hours.

• Echinacea can be used in whichever form you prefer, two or three times per day; see the guidelines on page 108. Do not continue this echinacea treatment for more than two consecutive weeks, as this intense usage can potentially work against your immune system if continued long-term (six to eight weeks).

• See Chapter 8 for specific symptom relief.

YOUR PLAN OF ATTACK IF A FLU VIRUS INVADES

The flu comes on fast and furious—usually within forty-eight hours of being exposed to the virus. The symptoms last for about a week. However, a dry cough and a feeling of fatigue can linger for several more weeks. The flu is not a new infection; it has been causing illness for a long time.

Each year, influenza outbreaks result in the deaths of approximately 20,000 Americans, and illness many times this amount. Historical accounts of illnesses matching the description of the flu suggest that influenza has been around for many centuries. Local epidemics continue to occur each year and, in some years, influenza spreads to become pandemic, affecting people all over the world. In fact, the influenza pandemic of 1917 to 1919 killed more people than did all of the fighting in World War I. We're not suggesting that a fatal wave of the flu will sweep your street, but we are communicating how powerful the flu virus is, and why it's important to do what you can to shield your body from its effects.

Although a flu vaccine is available at the beginning of every flu season (October to November), the vaccine does not ensure universal protection because it does not guard against every strain of the flu virus. This is one of the reasons why building your immunity and being aware of ways to reduce your exposure to infectious organisms is important. The advice for preventing the flu is the same as for preventing colds. Please refer this chapter's sections on lifestyle and diet advice for boosting immune function and preventing viral infections (pages 99 to 107).

If the flu has taken hold of you, there is action you can take to weaken the virus. You should seriously consider herbal remedies and enhanced supplement usage. The following herbs will help boost your immunity, so that you can fight off the flu more effectively: elderberry; ginseng; and green tea. Explanations and dosages of these herbs can be found in Chapter 6. Also be sure to keep taking your vitamins and minerals, especially vitamins C and E and zinc, as directed for general prevention earlier in this chapter.

The following hour-by-hour, day-by-day plan will ensure that either your symptoms are arrested or your bout with the flu is much easier to deal with. This supplement plan has the best chances of being effective the earlier you start. So pay close attention to your body and start this flu attack plan at the first moment you suspect a flu is coming on. You will notice that the flu plan is very similar to the cold plan, with some additions and minor changes. Don't forget to keep your home stocked with the most crucial supplements year-round, so that you can achieve the fastest response time.

IMMEDIATE ACTIONS

Oftentimes, you will not know by the initial symptoms whether you have the common cold, the flu, or perhaps a bacterial infection. Nevertheless, it's best that you immediately start the attack plan if you notice body aches, fatigue, fever and chills, or sore throat.

- Take 3 to 5 grams of vitamin C. You may wish to stock 500-milligram tablets/capsules and take six to ten of these.

- Allow a zinc lozenge—containing 10 to 23 milligrams of zinc in the form of zinc gluconate, zinc gluconate/ glycine, or zinc acetate—to dissolve in your mouth. It doesn't hurt to use a zinc lozenge right away, even if you're not sure that your vague symptoms will result in a flu. Keep this lozenge in your mouth for as long as you can, at a minimum of five to ten minutes. Swallowing the lozenge early will reduce the time necessary for the zinc to be absorbed into the tissues of the mouth and throat to kill viruses.

- Take one cup of elderberry tea, or take standardized elderberry liquid extract. A good extract dose is 10 milliliters for adults and 5 milliliters for children.

- Echinacea can be used in whichever form you prefer, either as a tea (1 gram to a cup); fluid extract (alcohol-, water-, or glycerin-based); or tincture, 3 to 5 milliliters (5 ml equals one teaspoon); capsules/tablets, 200 to 400 milligrams.

- Drink extra fluids. Water and herbal teas, such as peppermint, ginger, and chamomile, are great choices.

THE FIRST DAY

Over the first day of full-blown flu symptoms, follow these guidelines every two to three hours:

- Take 1 gram of vitamin C.

- Dissolve one zinc lozenge in your mouth. If symptoms are not improved, you can take a zinc lozenge as often as once every hour. One drawback to this frequent use is palate irritation.

- Alternate elderberry and echinacea; see the guidelines on page 112.

THE FIRST NIGHT

If your symptoms have persisted to bedtime, we recommend using the above therapy of vitamin C, zinc, elderberry, and echinacea immediately before you retire for the night. If you do happen to wake up in the middle of the night, at the least allow a zinc lozenge to melt in your mouth for a few minutes. We have found that even when symptoms are controlled the first day, if the flu virus is given a breather overnight, the symptoms could return by morning.

THE FOLLOWING DAYS

Over the next couple of days, until your symptoms resolve, continue drinking extra fluids. Rest if you feel fatigued, and use a humidifier if your nasal passages feel dry. Every three to four hours, do the following:

- Take 500 milligrams of vitamin C.

- Dissolve one zinc lozenge in your mouth (if you can tolerate it, take a zinc lozenge every 2 to 3 hours).

- Alternate elderberry and echinacea. Or you might consider mixing smaller amounts of these herbs, along with boneset, and taking this mixture several times daily.

- See Chapter 8 for specific symptom relief.

After three days, if you have not improved, please keep in close contact with your physician, particularly if you have a high fever, vomiting, green mucus, or marked lethargy, or if you are unable to maintain adequate fluid intake. Sometimes the symptoms of a bacterial infection can mimic those of the common cold or the flu. Also keep in mind that although nutritional and herbal therapies are very beneficial, they are not always curative and they can not always be relied on exclusively.

N-ACETYL-CYSTEINE (NAC) SUPPLEMENTATION

N-acetyl-cysteine, better known as NAC, is made from the amino acid cysteine. NAC is known to help break down mucus. An inhaled form of NAC is used in hospitals as a treatment for bronchitis. However, the capsules/tablets of NAC has also been researched for easing flulike symptoms.

A double-blind, six-month study involving 263 adults provided either 1,200 milligrams of NAC or a placebo daily (De Flora, 1997). During that time, the number of people who came down with the flu and the severity of their symptoms were tracked. Although a similar number of people in both groups were found to have the flu virus upon testing, 79 percent of the placebo group had noticeable symptoms, while only 25 percent of the NAC group exhibited outward symptoms. This means that many people in the NAC group had the flu, but they didn't suffer many symptoms. In addition, the NAC-treated folks who did have symptoms experienced less severe symptoms and spent less time in bed.

Certainly more research is needed before making wide recommendations for the use of NAC to prevent the flu. This nutrient is expensive and hence we recommend it in a lower dose of 600 milligrams, for temporary use only in susceptible or at-risk individuals. And these individuals should take it only during the height of the cold and flu season, during an epidemic, or when they know they have been exposed to the virus.

HOMEOPATHY AS ANOTHER OPTION

Homeopathy is a philosophy of healing that uses very small amounts of naturally occurring substances (of plant, mineral, or animal origin) to stimulate a person's own healing or protection from illness. Scientific studies with homeopathy have not often provided consistent results. However, many homeopaths report positive results with homeopathic preparations for colds and the flu, as well as other infections.

There has been one study that specifically focused on the flu (Ferley, 1989). This double-blind clinical trial compared a homeopathic remedy called oscillococcinum with a placebo in 478 individuals who had come down with the flu. Symptoms of fever, headache, stiffness, pain, chills, cough, and fatigue were recorded for a week. Approximately 17 percent of the oscillococcinum users recovered within the first 48 hours, while only 10 percent of the placebo group recovered in that time period.

We recommend that you should first try the nutritional and herbal approaches to treating your cold or flu. However, if these are not effective, the use of oscillococcinum is an option. See a homeopath or trained personnel at your health store for more information.

THE WAY TO KEEP YOUR KIDS COLD-FREE

The average child experiences six to eight colds each year. Colds are even more frequent in households with more than one small child. Furthermore, families whose children attend daycare get twice as many colds.

Many young children are given over-the-counter cold remedies. Such medications are either ineffective at the dosages that are safe for small children, or if used in higher dosages, can lead to potentially deadly side effects. For example, high doses of acetaminophen—a substance found in non-aspirin pain relievers such as Tylenol—can cause irreparable liver damage and even fatalities (Turow, 1997).

In addition, antibiotics are often used inappropriately for colds and have their own set of side effects, including nausea, vomiting, diarrhea, and possibly severe allergic reactions that lead to hospitalization and deaths. Adding further to this problem is the fact that seasonal allergies are often mistaken for cold symptoms in children. The underlying allergy should be diagnosed and addressed. Giving the child medications to relieve the symptoms will mask the problem; it does no help in the long-run. Natural remedies are best.

Healthy Lifestyle Habits for Children

The advice discussed for boosting the immune system in adults generally holds true for children. Children should eat a wholesome diet with plenty of fruits and vegetables, while limiting sugar (including sodas), as well as processed, fast, and high-fat foods. Plenty of fluids will keep their systems cleansed and hydrated. Kids should engage in physical activity, have adequate sleep habits, and be exposed to minimal stress, but maximal love and support in the family.

It is particularly important for kids to be reminded to wash their hands frequently, especially if the child or another family member currently has a cold. And children should be told not to share toothbrushes, eating utensils, or similar household items with their siblings.

Vitamin and Herbal Remedies for Children

Herbal remedies can generally be used for treating colds

and the flu in children. There are products available in pharmacies and health food stores that are specifically designed for children; follow the dosage information listed on the label. As a general rule, a safe amount of herbal remedies for children can be determined by dividing your child's weight in pounds by 150 and using the resulting fraction as a guide for what portion of the regular adult dose to give. For example, if your child weighs 50 pounds, one-third of the adult dose should be used. Since the adult dosage of echinacea is 900 milligrams total over the course of a day, the appropriate dosage for a 50-pound child would be 300 milligrams per day.

Liquid forms of natural remedies are often the best choice for kids. If using tinctures, choose the water- or glycerin-based tinctures, as opposed to the alcohol-based kinds. You can also try mixing powdered nutrients or herbs in foods such as applesauce, to make the supplements more palatable.

The administration of vitamin C to children has been reviewed. The results found that according to the ten placebo-controlled studies available, regular consumption of 1,000 milligrams of vitamin C alleviated the symptoms of the common cold, as evidenced by shorter cold duration and/or fewer missed days of school (Hemilä, 1997). Since children have difficulty swallowing pills, you can mix powdered vitamin C in juice or water. If your child is prone to colds, you may wish to provide 250 to 500 milligrams daily of vitamin C during the winter season. For the rest of the year, 50 to 100 milligrams daily should provide adequate supplementation. We do not recommend chewable vitamin C because it has been known to contribute to dental cavities.

The use of nutritional and herbal therapies are often effective in children. However, please keep a close eye on the symptoms to make sure that a more serious infection is not brewing or that your child is not having an adverse reaction to the therapy. In particular, consult your pediatrician if there is high fever, yellow or green mucus, vomiting, lethargy, or refusal to eat or drink.

What About Zinc Lozenges for Children?

The results of the first study that examined the potential of zinc lozenges in children and teenagers were not encouraging (Macknin, 1998). Approximately 250 students from first through twelfth grades were assigned to take either zinc lozenges or placebo lozenges. Each zinc lozenge supplied 10 milligrams of zinc in the zinc gluconate glycine form. Five to six lozenges were taken daily, starting within twenty-four hours of the first cold symptoms. By the end of the study, there was no significant difference between the groups in terms of how many days the children suffered from a variety of cold symptoms.

The are several reasons why this study might have failed. For starters, far fewer zinc lozenges were used in this study than in studies of adults that showed beneficial results. In addition, it is important to allow the zinc lozenge to completely dissolve in the mouth. Children might have quickly chewed and swallowed the lozenges, not giving the zinc the time and exposure to the mouth and throat areas that may be necessary to kill the viruses. It's also possible that many of the children had cold symptoms for longer than twenty-four hours by the time they related them to their parents or researchers.

Since there is excellent evidence that zinc in the form of lozenges can interfere with viral replication, we believe that zinc should be given an opportunity to be used in children who come down with cold symptoms, particularly for the first day or two. (The results of the one study discussed above are not conclusive enough yet to convince us otherwise.) However, remind your child to allow the zinc lozenge to dissolve completely, for at least five to ten minutes, and to use the zinc lozenges every hour or two during the first day of treatment. Some disadvantages of zinc are that it can cause soreness in the mouth and nausea if used frequently, and may be distasteful. Find a product in which the bitter taste of the zinc is well disguised.

THE NO-COLD KIT FOR TRAVELERS

Traveling greatly increases your risk of coming down with a cold. This is especially true if you are traveling by airplane, due to close proximity to fellow travelers, low humidity in the cabin, stress of travel, time change leading to jet lag, alterations in sleep patterns, changes in dietary habits, and so on. And if your flight is during the winter holiday season, you should take special heed to this section, since bugs are rampant and your immunity is probably less than perfect due to holiday stress. But there are ways to avoid getting sick from one of the many bugs lurking along your travel path. How do we know? Because we both travel frequently and have found personal success with the following plan.

The Three Days Prior to Your Travel

In preparing to travel, ensure that your diet is based on wholesome foods, especially fruits and vegetables. Incorporate garlic into your meals and consider drinking green tea in place of coffee or black tea. Also consider taking 1 gram of vitamin C, two or three times per day.

When You're on Your Way

Once your plane trip has begun, take a zinc lozenge and allow it to dissolve in your mouth. Take another gram of vitamin C. Continue to take this dose two or three times per day.

At Your Destination

Once you reach your place of destination, you can assist your immune system by following this advice. Take 0.5 to 2 milligrams of melatonin—a natural hormone that promotes sleep—about one to three hours before your new bedtime, to help you adjust to the new time zone, if necessary. The time-release form of melatonin is a good option. If you notice symptoms, continue taking vitamin C and zinc lozenges as recommended under "The Three Days Prior to Your Travel," for at least two days. Also in the case of symptoms, take echinacea two or three times per day. The appropriate dosage is: 1 cup of tea; 1 to 2 milliliters of fluid extract; 3 to 4 milliliters of tincture; or 200 to 400 milligrams in capsules/tablets.

Remember to bring along an ample supply of supplements in order to be prepared if you do catch a bug. Thus, you will minimize the impact it has on your vacation or business function. Also keep in mind that you may not be able to find a pharmacy or health food store at your destination, especially if you travel overseas.

CONCLUSION

By now it should be clear that you have a lot of "tools" for preventing and treating the common cold and the flu. By following the advice in this chapter, you'll greatly increase your chances of a cold-free, flu-free winter. And if you are invaded by a virus, you'll know how to stop that infection in its tracks. To further help you in targeting the discomforts that ail you most, the following chapter addresses individual symptoms and covers several natural remedies for each.

8 *Natural Remedies for Specific Symptoms*

W hen it comes to nursing yourself through an upper respiratory tract infection, the basics are of utmost importance: Get plenty of rest, drink lots of fluids, and eat healthy. But you also want to gain some relief from the specific symptoms that you experience. There are natural options to do so. The most frequently suffered cold and flu symptoms are listed alphabetically in this chapter, and natural remedies are suggested.

Many of the recommended natural remedies are herbal treatments. Please refer to Chapter 6 for information about the mentioned herbs, their forms and safety. Also, keep in mind that research with herbal therapies in treating symptoms of colds and flu is still in the early stages. Further scientific studies may confirm or dispute the early findings and the folkloric recommendations. Much of our knowledge comes from the traditional uses of these herbs and the experience of herbalists in their practices.

CONGESTION

During a cold or flu episode, feeling "stuffed up" often occurs after a runny nose. At first it's a relief to not be blowing your nose every few minutes, but struggling to breathe through blocked nostrils quickly becomes very frustrating. This symptom can even interfere with sleep. Although over-the-counter decongestants such as pseudoephedrine may do the most effective job of clearing congestion, some may cause insomnia and raise blood pressure. So below, we suggest natural decongestants to open clogged nasal passages and to dry profuse mucus. Keep in mind that it is very important to drink copious amounts of fluids during times of congestion, to flush out the system and keep cells hydrated.

Herbal Remedies

The following herbs are suggested treatments for relief from congestion:

Horseradish. If you don't mind spicy food, eating horseradish (the fresh root or prepared horseradish dressing) or the Japanese horseradish called wasabi provides temporary relief for stuffed sinuses. Lisa Alschuler, N.D., an expert in herbal therapy from Bastyr University in Seattle, Washington, recommends making a poultice of horseradish powder and applying it over the nose or sinuses. Horseradish can easily be obtained in a grocery store.

Ma Huang. Many over-the-counter decongestants contain ephedrine and pseudoephedrine—substances that are derived from the ma huang herb. Ma huang is effective for relieving nasal congestion. However, along with this action, it can raise blood pressure and lead to nervousness. When used later than mid-afternoon, it can even cause insomnia. It is prudent not to use this herb in children, and to use it cautiously (and in small amounts) in adults. If using substances that contain ephedrine, maximum daily dose should not exceed 30 milligrams of ephedrine; if using substances that contain pseudoephedrine, maximum daily dose should not exceed 120 milligrams of pseudo-ephedrine.

Mullein. This herb helps loosen and expel mucus and has the added benefit of soothing the sore throat that often accompanies congestion during a cold. Tea made from dried leaves or flowers is probably the best form of this herb, since warm liquids have other benefits when you have a sore throat.

Aromatic Oils of Herbs

Aromatic oils, such as the oils of eucalyptus, peppermint, and menthol, can be used as inhalants to ease nasal congestion. To use as an inhalant, combine the herbs with hot water in a bowl, cover your head with a towel, and smell the vapor.

Zinc

Several studies have documented the ability of zinc lozenges to help resolve a stuffy nose, although the effects can be mild (Godfrey, 1992). Zinc lozenges also help shorten the overall duration of a cold episode. Keep lozenges in the mouth as long as possible and take them frequently. If you wake up in the middle of the night during a cold, take another lozenge. (For more information, see Chapter 4.)

Other Natural Decongestants

To make saline nose drops, add half of a teaspoon of salt to two cups of warm water that has been boiled to rid it of chlorine and to sterilize it. (Chlorine can cause congestion.)

Another option is to use distilled water. Administer with a dropper, and use as needed to relieve nasal congestion. This technique helps to flush out the nasal passages.

And scientific research has confirmed what Mom knew all along: chicken soup is good for a cold. Why? Because it increases the flow of mucus from the nose (Saketkhoo, 1978).

COUGH

A cough is one of the most frequently occurring symptoms of the common cold, and it is often the last symptom of a cold or flu to go away. In such cases, because of irritation to the lungs, a dry cough continues. If the cough is not relieved after a few days, then your doctor may wish to prescribe you a temporary prescription cough suppressant and/or to determine if there's an underlying serious infection. As a last resort, some doctors prescribe codeine, or a short course (such as five to seven days) of a steroid such as prednisone, to halt the cough.

Please keep in mind that a cough is your body's natural way to expel mucus, and suppression is not always a good idea. However, if you have a dry, annoying cough that is making you miserable and interfering with sleep, then the following natural cough suppressants or expectorants can ease your symptom.

Herbal Remedies

For cough relief, try the following herbs:

Wild Cherry. The bark of this tree has a long tradition both as an expectorant (that is, to help expel mucus) and as a cough suppressant. It is commonly found as a syrup, but can also be drank in tea form; you can add honey, stevia, or lemon to improve its flavor. The effects are weak, so don't expect it to be as powerful as codeine.

Slippery Elm. This herb is another way to quell a cough because of the mucilage content. We've found slippery elm lozenges to be helpful for coughing episodes. Slippery elm can also act as a demulcent to soothe the throat, and as an expectorant. Herbalist Janet Zand finds slippery elm to be very useful in relieving cough symptoms.

Additional Herbs. Marshmallow and mullein contain mucilage, which is soothing for coughs. And echinacea and elderberry have been found to shorten the number of days of coughing during an infection (Degenring, 1995; Zakay-Rones, 1995).

You will find that many of the herbs recommended in this section are combined to make cough formulas. Alternatively, you can combine several of these herbs in a tea made at home, and drink a cup every few hours.

For a dry cough, Dr. Alschuler recommends licorice tea every few hours. In between, you can take myrrh tincture mixed in water. Dr. Alschuler also finds mullein to be helpful. Mullein can be combined in a tea form with licorice.

N-acetyl-cysteine (NAC)

Chris Meletis, N.D., Dean of Clinical Affairs and Chief Medical Officer at the National College of Naturopathic Medicine in Portland, Oregon, reports good success with temporarily using 600 milligrams of N-acetyl-cysteine, three times a day. The NAC acts as a mucolytic and expectorant. NAC is a good nutrient for respiratory tissues and is best suited for a productive cough with thick mucus. It helps to break up the mucus and also has antioxidant properties. For more information on NAC, see pages 114 to 115.

Other Natural Cough Suppressants and Expectorants

Sucking on hard candy, drinking tea (or similar warm beverages), and inhaling steam are other ways to ease a cough.

To help relieve coughs that bring up mucus, drink plenty of water to thin the mucus and use a humidifier to loosen it.

A honey/lemon mixture can be effective, as well. Mix two parts honey with one part lemon juice. The honey is soothing to the throat, and also acts as an expectorant. Some studies have found that honey has antiviral activities (Zeina, 1996). The lemon juice helps reduce the thickness of the phlegm. Adults can take this mixture by the teaspoonful, as needed. Children should take only a quarter of a teaspoon, used cautiously as needed. Do not give honey to infants under one year of age.

FATIGUE

Fatigue is a message from your body; it tells you to take it easy. When you feel fatigued, the best thing to do is to rest and to allow healing to take place. Along with a feeling of fatigue, many people find that they are slightly depressed. This is particularly true during the flu. It is believed that certain substances released by the immune system, such as cytokines, are able to go to the brain and interfere with the proper functioning of brain chemicals, including serotonin, which contributes to low mood.

When the flu drags on for a few days, it can feel interminable. Try to keep up a positive attitude and remind yourself that the feelings of tiredness and depression are not permanent. Eventually your infection will be over and you will recover your full energy and vitality. Make sure, though, that you keep up your fluid intake. Soups and teas are great options. Furthermore, eat small amounts of foods throughout the day.

Your Herbal and Vitamin/Mineral Regimens

Your energy will return a little more during each day of your recovery. Although natural stimulants, such as ginseng, are known to increase energy, their use is not recommended during a cold or flu. *If you were taking tonics such as ginseng, astragalus, reishi, and other herbs before your infection, it's time that you take a break from their use.* Your body wants to rest and take naps. Being on a stimulant may interfere with your body's need to relax.

However, we do encourage that you continue taking your multivitamin/mineral and B vitamins. For example, a healthy regimen is to take a moderate-dose, "one-a-day" formulation and a B-complex supplement. The B vitamins can provide energy.

Melatonin—A Natural Sleep Enhancer

Fatigue can be aggravated by a disturbance in the sleep cycle and lack of adequate sleep. Hence, consider taking melatonin at a dose of 0.3 to 1.0 milligram on an empty stomach, about an hour or two before bed, for two to three nights. This will help you get a deeper sleep. Please keep in mind, though, that excess melatonin, such as more than 1 or 2 milligrams, can make you sleepier during the day.

FEVER

Fever is one of your body's ways to fight an infection. The body's intent in raising temperature is to make it a more difficult and hostile environment for the invading bugs. Therefore, fever, up to a certain degree, is beneficial and could slow cold and flu virus proliferation.

In most healthy individuals, normal body temperature ranges between 96.6°F (36.0°C) and 99.0°F (37.2°C). Body temperature is lowest in the middle of night, between 2 and 4 A.M., while it is highest in the early evening, between 6 and 10 P.M. Body temperature rarely exceeds 102°F during a cold. So, the use of fever-reducing medicines is rarely required. However, during the flu, body temperature can rise as high as 105°F. These high levels are very uncomfortable. Therefore, it is important to find some relief. There is no need to lower temperature all the way back down to normal. The intent is to make the fever tolerable.

We strongly advise that you keep in touch with your health-care provider anytime you have a high fever, particularly if it persists or is associated with vomiting or difficulty in retaining fluids. Fever can often be due to bacterial infections. Sometimes there can be a superimposed infection on top of a cold or flu. This means that the infection initially started out as a simple cold or flu, but bacteria found the opportunity to also get involved and worsen the infection into more severe conditions, such as pneumonia or bacterial pharyngitis.

We recommend that you do not treat a mild fever right away. However, if you are uncomfortable, you can try one of the following natural fever reducers. As a rule, the teas work well, although you can also try the tinctures or pills.

Herbal Remedies

The following herbs are effective in treating fever:

Boneset. This Native American herb was used traditionally to treat fevers associated with colds and the flu, particularly if the fever was accompanied by aches and pains. Boneset can be drank as a tea, several times per day. The taste of boneset is terrible, and hence you may wish to combine it with a small amount of honey or sweeten it with the natural sweetener stevia.

White Willow and Meadowsweet. White willow is the parent material from which aspirin is derived. Like aspirin (a stronger substance), white willow lowers fevers. Willow bark extracts containing salicin—a compound chemically related to aspirin—are available as capsules. Another herb that contains salicin is meadowsweet. Interestingly, meadowsweet also contains substances similar to the blood thinner heparin (Liapina, 1993; Kudriashov, 1991).

Children and people who are allergic to aspirin should not use white willow or meadowsweet, nor should those younger than age fourteen. Also, white willow and meadowsweet are not as powerful as aspirin in lowering fever or reducing aches and pains. Please keep in mind that the amount of salicin found in white willow and meadowsweet are much less that what you would get if you ingested aspirin itself. These herbs will not have the same power punch as taking a 325-milligram pill of aspirin.

Other Natural Fever Reducers

Herbalists Kilham and Smith both report yarrow to be an additional herb helpful in reducing fever. Making yarrow tea, notes Kilham, is not only great for bringing down a fever, but it also clears congestion. Also, try a lukewarm or slightly cool bath if you need to temporarily reduce fever.

NAUSEA

Nausea, the very uncomfortable sensation that you are going to vomit, and stomach upset are much more common with the flu than a cold. There are steps you can take to relieve this miserable feeling.

Ginger

The herb ginger has been well-tested for its anti-nausea properties when it comes to motion sickness, and this effect probably holds true for nausea associated with other conditions, such as the flu (Grontved, 1988). Teas are fine, but tinctures and capsules/tablets have been found to be much more effective.

Dietary Advice

If your nausea has progressed to vomiting, try the following suggestions. Keep away from food for one hour. If nothing else will stay down, at least suck on ice chips or popsicles to avoid dehydrating. A good remedy is to sip on lukewarm cola that has been "defizzed." This not only helps to control the nausea, but also provides sugar and potassium.

As you improve, include soup, diluted fruit juices, bouillon, gelatin, bananas, crackers, or applesauce in your diet. Also, peppermint helps quell muscle spasms in the digestive tract, and can help during nausea and vomiting. Peppermint tea would be a tasty way to use this herb. Other herbs with soothing effects on the gastrointestinal tract include chamomile and lemon balm.

MUSCLE ACHES, HEADACHES, AND OTHER PAIN

Pain, most often headaches and muscle aches, is a common symptom during viral infections, particularly during the flu virus. Aches and pains can be felt in most muscle groups, including the arms, legs, and the lower back. Patients also report a dull pain or pressure in back of the eyes.

As a rule, herbal pain relievers are not as powerful as aspirin, acetaminophen, codeine, and non-steroidal anti-inflammatory drugs like ibuprofen or naproxen. However, side effects and risks from herbal treatments are less common and less severe. For starters, aspirin should not be given to children under the age of fourteen when treating colds, since it is associated with the rare neurological condition known as Reye's syndrome.

Although small amounts of acetaminophen are safe, overdoses are common each year, causing liver damage and fatalities. Since acetaminophen is contained in many

When Should I Call a Doctor?

Cold and flu symptoms can be eased or relieved with the natural remedies outlined in this chapter, but contact your physician if the symptoms listed below are present. Also, keep in close contact with your physician if you have an infant or young child who is suffering from a cold or flu. The safety of most of the remedies in this book have not specifically been evaluated in infants.

Throat

- Your throat is sore for more than forty-eight hours.

- The inside of your throat is beefy-red (not just pinkish-red), swollen, and pus-covered.

- You've been exposed to someone who has strep throat (a bacterial infection).

- You have a red rash that feels likes sandpaper. (This could mean a bacterial strep throat).

Nose and Head

- You have a runny nose for more than ten days.

- Your nasal discharge is yellow or green and lasts all day long.

- You have severe facial pain or headache.

Cough

- Your cough lasts longer than seven days.

- Your coughing is severe; or it hurts to cough; or coughing produces thick, rusty, or greenish mucus.

- You have chest pain when you breathe, or you have difficulty breathing through your mouth.

Ears

- You have severe pain in your ear.

- You have discharge from your ear.

- Your ears are still bothering you after seven days.

Fever

- You have a temperature of 102°F or greater.

- Your fever lasts more than four days.

- You have shaking chills, soaking sweats, shortness of breath, or mental confusion.

- A fever of over 101°F begins after the third day of your illness.

Abdomen and Gastrointestinal Tract

- You have persistent pain in your abdomen or rectum, or if pain is localized in one area of your abdomen.

- You have black or bloody stools or vomit, or there is a "coffee grounds" appearance to your vomit.

- You have more than eight bowel movements per day.

These are general guidelines. You know yourself best. And if you are a parent, you know your child best. If the illness is very worrisome, or if you feel (or your child looks) very sick, call your doctor, regardless of how long the symptoms have been occurring or how common they may sound.

over-the-counter cold formulas, overdoses occur when parents mistakenly give excessive amounts to infants and small children. In addition, one Australian study with college students has indicated that using aspirin or acetaminophen during a cold may suppress the immune response, increase the number of days of viral shedding, and slightly worsen runny nose and nasal congestion (Graham, 1990). But in cases of severe aches and pains that do not respond to the herbal therapies, the cautious and temporary use of pharmaceutical medicines is justified.

Herbal Remedies

Try using the following herbs for pain relief:

Boneset. This Native American herb was used traditionally to treat fevers associated with colds and flu, particularly if the fever was accompanied by aches and pains. Boneset tea can be drunk several times a day. The taste of boneset is terrible, and hence you may wish to combine it with a small amount of honey or sweeten it with stevia.

Red Pepper. Capsaicin, the ingredient in red pepper that makes it taste hot, is a pain reliever. Taken in capsule/tablet form, red pepper might help ease your headaches or muscle aches during an infection.

White Willow and Meadowsweet. Both of these herbs contain salicin, a close cousin to aspirin. The pain-relieving and fever-lowering effects of these herbs are not as powerful as aspirin, but their use can help take the edge off your aches. It's best that those allergic to aspirin and children younger than age fourteen not take these herbs.

Other Natural Pain Relievers

A warm bath, especially with Epsom salts, can comfort achy muscles. Actually, you can find many powdered salts of sodium and magnesium in your local drug store. They can be added to warm bath-water to contribute to a soothing soak.

Sometimes pain can interfere with sleep. In this situation, to help you reach a deeper, more restorative sleep, use melatonin (see page 127).

RUNNY NOSE

Most colds and even the flu start out with thin, watery discharge from the nose that later thickens to cause congestion. But more vexing than the nasal discharge itself is the irritation that can accompany constant nose-running, -rubbing, and -blowing. Just a few days after the start of your runny nose, you could well begin to look like Rudolph the Red-Nosed Reindeer.

The temptation during this time is to rush to the pharmacy to purchase over-the-counter nasal drops. The medicines found in these nasal drops most commonly include phenylephrine or oxymetazoline. We strongly recommend that you do not use nasal drops or sprays that contain decongestants. Although they are effective in temporarily stopping the runny nose, you soon pay the piper. The runny nose and/or congestion returns more viciously and tolerance to the medicines can develop. The return and aggravation of these symptoms is called the "rebound effect." The only time we would acquiesce to the use of nose drops is when you are in bed and the runny nose is making it impossible for you to fall asleep.

We also strongly recommend you avoid the use of antihistamines, such as diphenhydramine, since their use is more appropriate for allergic symptoms and not for symptoms due to viral infections. But do keep up your fluid intake by drinking plenty of warm liquids. Herbal and nutritional options to decreasing or stopping symptoms of runny nose are limited. But consider that a runny nose is your body's way to get rid of viruses. Hence, it is not necessary to completely eliminate the runny nose—just control it enough to make you feel comfortable and to avoid spending a week's wages on tissues.

Herbal Remedies

The following herbal treatments are helpful for the relief of a runny nose:

Ma Huang. This herb is the most effective herb for stopping a runny nose. Many over-the-counter decongestants contain ephedrine, pseudoephedrine, or related chemicals. These chemicals are extracted or based on the ma huang herb.

While ma huang is effective for relieving nasal congestion, it can raise blood pressure and lead to insomnia, restlessness, and nervousness. It is prudent to not use this herb in children, and to use it cautiously and in small amounts in adults. If using a substance that contains ephedrine, maximum daily dosage should not exceed 30 milligrams of ephedrine; if using a substance that contains pseudoephedrine, maximum daily dosage should not exceed 120 milligrams of pseudoephedrine. It's best not to take any decongestant past 4 P.M., in order to avoid insomnia.

Echinacea. There is evidence that echinacea shortens the number of days you'll have a runny nose after you've caught a cold. Researchers actually documented this by counting how many tissues cold victims used (Scaglione, 1995). If you have a cold or flu, chances are you are already taking echinacea. (For more information, see Chapter 5.) But we also strongly recommend it for this specific symptom.

Zinc

Zinc lozenges were reported to help people recover more quickly from colds—especially from the symptom of a runny nose (Godfrey, 1992; Mossad, 1996). In part, the astringency of zinc remedies a runny nose because it dries out the nasal passages. Another contributing factor might be that zinc temporarily (for about one to three hours) interferes with nerve impulses that are involved in nasal discharge (Novick, 1997).

Other Natural Remedies

Putting face cream or aloe vera lotion around the outside of the nostrils can reduce the chafing caused by blowing the nose.

SORE THROAT

A scratchy or sore throat is generally the earliest symptom of an impending cold infection. However, this same symptom can be the beginning of a strep throat—a bacterial infection that requires antibiotics. During the early symptoms, even experienced doctors sometimes have difficulty determining whether a sore throat is caused by a virus or a bacteria. Both types of infections can cause fever and malaise. Although fever is generally higher in bacterial throat infections, look for additional symptoms that can differentiate the two; it is rare for bacterial infections to be associated with a runny nose or nasal congestion. Regardless of whether it is a bacterial or viral infection, the following natural remedies can go a long way towards providing you the relief you seek for a painful throat.

Herbal Remedies

Most of the herbs discussed in this section have demulcent properties—they help soothe a sore throat. Some of them contain mucilage, a thick substance that helps relieve discomfort. These herbs are most effective as lozenges, syrups, or as teas, especially if you are able to gargle with the tea. You can often find these herbs in various combinations.

Echinacea. Aside from shortening the length of your infection, echinacea might help you get over a sore throat caused by a cold or flu. Studies have shown that this herb helps to relieve the discomfort of this symptom (Degenring, 1995; Braunig, 1992). See Chapter 5 for detailed information on echinacea.

Licorice. This herb has been used for centuries to comfort the irritated throat during a cold. It is available as a tea, spray, and as an ingredient in lozenges. These forms allow direct contact with the throat tissues. Swallowing a capsule is not an effective way to take licorice for a sore throat.

Marshmallow. This herb is effective for soothing irritated mucous membranes, including those of the mouth and throat. You can drink it as a tea, or it can be found as an ingredient in lozenges and syrups.

Mullein. If a dry cough leads to throat irritation, mullein's mucilage content can help soothe the irritated mucous membranes in the throat.

Slippery Elm. Our first choice for a sore throat is slippery elm. It soothes the pain and irritation, providing temporary relief. This herb is frequently found in many cold preparations—in lozenges, teas, syrups, tinctures, and even as popsicles for children.

Zinc

A zinc lozenge, among its other benefits during a cold, can temporarily ease a sore throat. Patients often report that symptoms of sore throat are relieved within an hour of using the lozenge, and symptoms return if another is not taken within two to three hours. For the greatest effect, keep the zinc lozenge in your mouth as long as you can, for a minimum of ten minutes. However, if zinc lozenges irritate your mouth and palate, you are simply trading one pain for another and should reduce the frequency of use. (For more information, see Chapter 4.)

Other Natural Throat Soothers

To make a saline gargle, which is very soothing, add half of a teaspoon of salt to two cups of warm water. Gargle with this mixture as needed. Drinking warm tea also has a comforting effect on an irritated throat.

A WORD OF CAUTION

When used as directed, herbal remedies are generally safe. However, certain herbs can undesirably interact with specific over-the-counter and/or prescription drugs. So, if you are using any medication, it is important to inform your physician about which herbs you are also taking.

CONCLUSION

Research with herbs and nutrients to treat the symptoms of colds and flu is limited. Please keep in mind that most of our information is based on traditions and anecdotes. We certainly hope that more research will be conducted over the next few years regarding natural therapies for the common cold and the flu. In the meantime, it is nice to know that there are natural, safe ways to find symptom relief. There is little doubt that the use of herbs and nutrients can minimize your reliance on pharmaceutical cold medicines. We sincerely hope the suggestions in this chapter will lessen your winter misery.

Conclusion

An old saying goes, "A cold lasts seven days, but with proper treatment it can be shortened to last a week." The information in *The Common Cold Cure*, particularly the step-by-step guide presented in Chapter 7, challenges such an outdated belief. This book has covered natural ways to prevent and treat a cold or flu attack. Armed with these options, you can avoid the myriad of side effects that come pack-and-parcel with over-the-counter and prescription medications.

We do have one caution: If your symptoms do not improve within a brief period using natural therapies, please keep in close contact with your physician, particularly if you have a high fever, vomiting, green mucus, marked lethargy, or if you are unable to maintain adequate fluid intake. Sometimes the symptoms of a bacterial infection can mimic those of the common cold or the flu. Also keep in mind that although nutritional and herbal therapies are very beneficial, realistically they are not always curative and they cannot be relied on exclusively.

Our objective in this book has been to provide you with the latest research regarding the natural therapy of mild infection. Our hope is that the use of these therapeutic methods will decrease unnecessary office visits and the number of unnecessary prescriptions written for antibiotics during the treatment of colds and the flu.

After thoroughly reviewing a number of studies over the past few decades, regarding nutritional prevention of and therapy for minor infections, and after reviewing the traditional herbal remedies, we are convinced that this type of information should be presented to the public and to more doctors. In particular, those involved in family practice, pediatrics, and internal medicine should be aware of this information. We truly believe that if you follow the suggestions offered in *The Common Cold Cure*, you will avoid the majority of potential cold infections that could make you miserable.

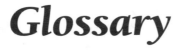

Glossary

Alkaloid—any of the hundreds of compounds, found in plants, with a nitrogen atom connected to two carbon atoms and often formed in a ring structure. Many commonly known chemicals and drugs are alkaloids, including nicotine, cocaine, quinine, morphine, and ephedrine.

Analgesic—a drug that reduces or takes away pain.

Antibody—a protein produced by the immune system in response to an antigen. It has the capacity to neutralize a specific antigen.

Antioxidant—a substance that combines with damaging molecules, neutralizes them, and thus prevents the deterioration of DNA, RNA, lipids, and proteins. Antioxidants are especially recognized as cancer-prevention agents. Vitamins C, E, and beta-carotene are the best known antioxidants, but more are being discovered every year.

Ayurveda—a traditional Hindu system of medicine practiced in India since the first century A.D. In treating diseases, Ayurvedic practitioners combine herbs, oils, and other natural remedies. Many herbs used in Ayurveda are now gaining popularity in Western countries.

B cell—a type of white blood cell that matures in the bone marrow (hence, the letter "B"). B cells are part of the immune system and circulate in the blood, constantly on the alert for invading germs.

Bacteria—single-celled microorganisms. Some cause disease, while others are harmless or even beneficial to biological processes.

Bone marrow—the soft material filling the inside of bone cavities. The bone marrow produces blood and immune cells.

Cell—the smallest organized unit of living structure in the body. There are trillions of cells in humans. In fact, the brain alone has close to one trillion cells.

Cortisol—also called hydrocortisone; a sterol (related to a steroid) secreted by the human adrenal glands. It is often released in high amounts during stress. High doses lead to interference with the proper functioning of the immune system.

Cytokine—hormone-like small proteins secreted by the immune system.

Demulcent—a medicine or ointment that soothes irritated or inflamed mucous membranes.

Double-blind study—a research study in which neither the researchers nor the volunteers know which participants are taking the medicine and which participants are taking the placebo until the code is broken at the end of the study.

Expectorant—a substance that helps to bring up phlegm or mucus from the lungs and bronchi.

Flavonoids—a class of phytonutrients that have antioxidant, anti-bacterial, anti-viral, and anti-allergic properties.

Flu—*see Influenza.*

Free radicals—highly reactive compounds that damage cell membranes and other cell components, contributing to degenerative diseases such as heart disease, cancer, premature aging, cataracts, arthritis, and many other conditions. They are found in air pollution, tobacco smoke, some foods, pesticides, and ultraviolet radiation. Free radicals are also manufactured during normal body processes.

Immune globulins—also called immunoglobulins; a group of proteins found in blood. Immune globulins fight off infections by attaching to and killing bacteria and viruses. The best known is gamma globulin.

Immune system—the body's system of resistance to disease that is provided by many specialized organs, tissues, and chemicals that work together.

Influenza—also called the flu; a virus infection causing symptoms similar to the common cold, but more serious. In fact, serious cases can lead to severe complications and even death.

Interferons—small proteins, produced by white blood cells, that fight some forms of cancer and infections, especially viral infections.

Leukocytes—term referring to the entire class of white blood cells.

Lymphocyte—a type of white blood cell that fights infections. Two major types are B lymphocytes (B cells) and T lymphocytes (T cells).

Macrophage—a large immune system cell that has the ability to be phagocytic—that is, to engulf and kill germs.

Macrophages are thought to be involved in plaque formation in arteries.

Microorganisms—bacteria, viruses, and other minute life forms that are only visible through a microscope. Many of these cause infections.

Minerals—inorganic (not produced by animals or plants) substances such as calcium and magnesium, many of which are essential for health.

Natural killer cell—a type of white blood cell that can destroy certain cancer cells and germs.

Phagocyte—a white blood cell that engulfs and ingests a harmful microorganism or substance in the blood stream, the skin, or other body tissues and organs.

Phytonutrients—non-nutritive, but health-enhancing compounds derived from many plant sources. The two major classes include carotenoids and flavonoids.

Placebo—a pill containing no active ingredients; a "dummy pill."

Placebo-controlled study—a study in which one group of volunteers takes a medicine or active treatment, while another group, called the control group, takes placebos. The results are compared to see how effective the medicine is.

Platelet—a small, round, or oval cell found in the blood and involved in blood clotting.

Polysaccharide—any of a group of complex carbohydrates having multiple single sugars attached to form long chains. Starch is a polysaccharide, as are countless combinations of different sugars. Some of these polysaccharides have immune-enhancing properties.

RDA (Recommended Daily Allowance)—a nutritional guideline for the appropriate doses of different vitamins and minerals required for good health. They are proposed by the Food and Drug Administration. Some scientists think that ingesting more than the RDA for certain nutrients may provide additional health benefits.

Saponins—compounds of plant origin that have the properties of foaming in water and of breaking up cell membranes.

Synergy—The increased effectiveness of herbs in combination, as opposed to the effectiveness of each herb taken individually.

T cell—a type of white blood cell that matures in the thymus gland (hence, the letter "T"). T cells are part of the immune system and constantly patrol the body for foreign matter and cancer cells.

Thymus gland—a gland that is located in the chest and participates in the production of white blood cells.

Tonic—an herb that increases energy levels and feelings of vitality.

Virus—a submicroscopic bug that can cause infection. Colds, flu, and AIDS are caused by viruses. Viruses cannot reproduce without a host body, and so are not technically considered to be independently living. Antibiotics cannot kill viruses.

Vitamins—essential nutrients found in foods. They are required only in minute amounts, but are absolutely necessary for proper body function. There are two classes of vitamins: water-soluble, such as vitamin C, and fat-soluble, such as vitamin E.

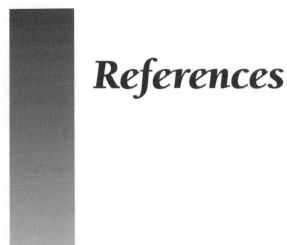

References

Chapter 1: Boost Your Immune System and Beat the Bugs

Barker, R., J. Burton, and P. Ziove, eds. *Principles of Ambulatory Medicine*, 3d ed. Baltimore, MD: Williams and Wilkins, 1991

Cohen, S., et al. "Types of stressors that increase susceptibility to the common cold in healthy adults," *Health Psychology* 17(3) (May 1998): 214–223.

Challem, J. *Beating the Supergerms*. New York, NY: Pocket Books, 1997.

Hayek, M.G., et al. "Vitamin E supplementation decreases lung virus titers in mice infected with influenza," *Journal of Infectious Diseases* 17 (1997): 273–276.

Huston, D. "The biology of the immune system," *Journal of the American Medical Association* 278 (1997): 1804–1814.

Chapter 2: Conventional Medicine Versus the Common Cold

Belshe, R., et al. "Intranasal flu vaccine," *New England Journal of Medicine* 338 (20) (1998): 1405–1412.

Cunningham, B, et al. "Viral upper respiratory tract infections in adults," *Institute for Clinical Systems Integration, Postgraduate Medicine* (Jan 1998): 71–80.

Makela, M.J., et al. "Viruses and bacteria in the etiology of the common cold," *Journal of Clinical Microbiology* 36(2) (Feb 1998): 539–542.

Niederman, M., et al. "Antibiotics or not? Managing patients with respiratory infections," *Patient Care* (Jan 15, 1998): 60–90.

Nyquist, A.C., et al. "Antibiotic prescribing for children with colds, upper respiratory tract infections, and bronchitis," *Journal of the American Medical Association* 279 (11) (1998): 875–882.

Smith, M., and W. Feldman. "Over-the-counter cold medication: A critical review of clinical trials between 1950 and 1991," *Journal of the American Medical Association* 269(17) (1993): 2258–2263.

Chapter 3: Vitamin C—Gold Medal Infection Fighter

Asfora, J. "Vitamin C in high doses in the treatment of the common cold," *International Journal for Vitamin and Nutrition Research* 16 (1977): 219–234.

Blanchard, J., M. Rowland, and T.N. Tozer. "Pharmacokinetic perspectives on megadoses of ascorbic acid," *American Journal of Clinical Nutrition* 66 (1997): 1061–1062.

Cathcart, R.F. "Vitamin C, titrating to bowel tolerance, anascorbemia, and acute induced scurvy," *Medical Hypotheses* 7 (1981): 1359–1376.

Cohen, H.A., H. Nahum, and I. Neuman. "Blocking effect of vitamin C in exercise-induced asthma," *Archives of Pediatric Medicine* 151 (1997): 367–370, 371.

Hemilä, H. "Does vitamin C alleviate the symptoms of the common cold? A review of current evidence," *Scandinavian Journal of Infectious Diseases* 26 (1994): 1–6.

Hemilä, H, and Z.S. Herman. "Vitamin C and the common cold: A restrospective analysis of Chalmers' review," *Journal of the American College of Nutrition* 14 (1995): 116–123.

Hemilä, H. "Vitamin C and common cold incidence: a review of studies with subjects under heavy physical stress," *International Journal of Sports Medicine* 17 (1996): 379–383.

Hemilä, H. "Vitamin C, the placebo effect, and the common cold: a case study of how preconceptions influence the analysis of results," *Journal of Clinical Epidemiology* 49 (1996): 1079–1084.

Hemilä, H. "Vitamin C intake and susceptibility to the common cold," *British Journal of Nutrition* 77 (1997): 59–72.

Hemilä, H. "Vitamin C intake and susceptibility to pneumonia," *Pediatric Infectious Disease Journal* 16 (1997): 836–837.

Hennet, T., E. Peterhans, and R. Stocker. "Alterations in antioxidant defences in lung and liver of mice infected with influenza A virus," *Journal of General Virology* 73 (1992): 39–46.

Hunt, C., et al. "The clinical effect of vitamin C supplementation in elderly hospitalised patients with acute respiratory infections," *Internation Journal for Vitamin and Nutrition Research* 64 (1994): 212–219.

Johnston, C.S., C. Corte, and E. Solomon. "Vitamin C status of a campus population: College students get a C minus," *Journal of the American College of Health* 46 (1998): 209–213.

Levine, M., et al. "Vitamin C pharmacokinetics in healthy volunteers: evidence for a recommended dietary allowance," *Proceedings of the National Academy of Sciences* 93 (1996): 3704–3709.

Podmore, I.D., et al. "Vitamin C exhibits pro-oxidant properties," *Nature* 392 (1998): 569.

Sapozhnikov, I.V., et al. "Nonspecific methods of prophylaxis of influenza and other acute respiratory diseases with dibasole and ascorbic acid," *Voprosy Virusologii* 4 (1976) 429–431.

Chapter 4: Zinc—A Cold's Worst Enemy

Douglas, R.M., et al. "Failure of effervescent zinc acetate lozenges to alter the course of upper respiratory tract infections in Australian adults," *Antimicrobial Agents and Chemotherapy* 31 (1987): 1263–1265.

Eby, G.A., D.R. Davis, and W.W. Halcomb. "Reduction in duration of common colds by zinc gluconate lozenges in a double-blind study," *Antimicrobial Agents and Chemotherapy* 25 (1984): 20–24.

Eby, G.A. "Zinc ion availability—the determinant of efficacy in zinc lozenge treatment of common colds," *Journal of Antimicrobial Chemotherapy* 40 (1997): 483–493.

Garland, M.L., K.O. Hagmeyer. "The role of zinc lozenges in treatment of the common cold," *Annals of Pharmacotherapy* 32 (1998): 63–69.

Godfrey, J.C., et al. "Zinc gluconate and the common cold: a controlled clinical study," *Journal of International Medical Research* 20 (1992): 234–236.

Macknin, M.L., et al. "Zinc gluconate lozenges for treating the common cold in children," *Journal of the Amercian Medical Association* 279 (1998): 1962–1967.

Marshall, S. "Zinc gluconate and the common cold. Review of randomized controlled trials," *Canadian Family Physician* 44 (1998): 1037–1042.

Mossad, S.B., et al. "Zinc gluconate lozenges for treating the common cold," *Annals of Internal Medicine* 125 (1996): 81–88.

Novick, S.G., et al. "How does zinc modify the common cold?" *Medical Hypotheses* 46 (1996): 295–302.

Novick, S.G., et al. "Zinc induced suppression of inflammation in the respiratory tract, caused by infection with human rhinovirus and other irritants," *Medical Hypotheses* 49 (1997): 347–357.

Ozturk, G., et al. "Decreased natural killer (NK) cell activity in zinc-deficient rats," *General Pharmacology* 25(7) (1994): 1499–1503.

Schlesinger, L., et al. "Zinc supplementation impairs monocyte function," *Acta Paediatrica* 82 (1993): 734–738.

Smith, D.S., et al. "Failure of zinc gluconate in treatment of acute upper respiratory tract infections," *Antimicrobial Agents and Chemotherapy* 33 (1989): 646–648.

Weismann, K., et al. "Zinc gluconate lozenges for common cold. A double-blind clinical trial," *Danish Medical Bulletin* 37 (1990): 279–281.

Zarembo, J.E., J.C. Godfrey, and N.J. Godfrey. "Zinc(II) in saliva: determination of concentrations produced by different formulations of zinc gluconate lozenges containing common excipients," *Journal of Pharmaceutical Sciences* 81 (1992): 128–130.

Chapter 5: Echinacea—Herbal Immune Activator

Bauer, R. "Echinacea drugs—effects and active ingredients," *Zeitschrift fur Arztliche Fortbildung* 90 (1996): 111–115.

Bauer, V.R., et al. "Immunologic in vivo and in vitro studies on Echinacea extracts," *Arzneimittel-Forschung* 38 (1988): 276–281.

Braunig, B., et al. "*Echinacea purpurea* root for strengthening the immune response in flu-like infection," *Zeitschrift fuer Phytotherapie* 13 (1992): 7–13.

Brown, D. *Herbal Prescriptions for Better Health.* Rocklin, CA: Prima Publishing, 1996.

Coeugniet, E.G., and E. Elek. "Immunomodulation with Viscum album and Echinacea purpurea extracts," *Onkologie* 10 (1987) 27–33

Combest, W., and G. Nemecz. "Echinacea," *U.S. Pharmacist* (Oct 1997).

Degenring, F.H. "Studies on the therapeutic efficacy of Echinaforce®." *Ganzheits Medizin* 2 (1995): 88–94.

Hobbs, C. *Echinacea. The Immune Herb!* Capitola, CA: Botanica Press, 1990.

Hobbs, C. "Echinacea: A literature review," *HerbalGram* 30 (1994): 33–48.

Leuttig, B., et al. "Macrophage activation by the polysaccharide arabinogalactan isolated from plant cell cultures of *Echinacea purpurea*," *Journal of the National Cancer Institute* 81 (1989): 669–675.

Melchart, D., et al. "Echinacea Root Extracts for the Prevention of Upper Respiratory Tract Infections: A Double-Blind, Placebo-Controlled Randomized Trial," *Archives of Family Medicine* 7 (1998): 541–545.

Melchart, D., et al. "Results of five randomized studies on the immunomodulatory activity of preparations of Echinacea," *Journal of Alternative and Complementary Medicine* 1 (1995): 145–160.

Mengs, U., C.B. Clare, and J.A. Poiley. "Toxicity of *Echinacea purpurea*. Acute, subacute and genotoxicity studies," *Arzneimittel-Forschung* 41 (1991): 1076–1081.

Mullins, R.J. "Echinacea-associated anaphylaxis," *Medical Journal of Australia* 168 (1998): 170–171.

Perry, N.B., et al. "Alkamide levels in *Echinacea purpurea*: A rapid analytical method revealing differences among roots, rhizomes, stems, leaves, and flowers," *Planta Medica* 63 (1997): 58–62.

Roesler, J., et al. "Application of purified polysaccharides from cell cultures of the plant *Echinacea purpurea* to test subjects mediates activation of the phagocyte system," *International Journal of Immunopharmacology* 13 (1991): 931–941.

Roesler, J., et al. "Application of purified polysaccharides from cell cultures of the plant *Echinacea purpurea* to mice mediates protection against systemic infections with Listeria monocytogenes and *Candida albicans*," *International Journal of Immunopharmacology* 13 (1991): 27–37.

Scaglione, F., and B. Lund. "Efficacy in the treatment of the common cold of a preparation containing an echinacea extract," *International Journal of Immunotherapy* 11 (1995): 163–166.

Schoenberger, D. "The influence of immune-stimulating effects of pressed juice from *Echinacea purpurea* on the course and severity of colds," *Forum Immunologie* 8 (1992): 2–12.

Steinmuller, C., et al. "Polysaccharides isolated from plant cell cultures of *Echinacea purpurea* enhance the resistance of immunosuppressed mice against systemic infections with *Candida albicans* and Listeria monocytogenes," *International Journal of Immunopharmacology* 15 (1993): 605–614.

Tubaro, A., et al. "Anti-inflammatory activity of a polysaccharidic fraction of Echinacea angustifolia," *Journal of Pharmacy and Pharmacology* 39 (1987): 567–569.

Tyler, V. *The Honest Herbal*, 3d ed. Binghamton, NY: Hawthorn Press, 1993.

Wagner, H., K. Jurcic. "Immunologic studies of plant combination preparations. In-vitro and in-vivo studies on the stimulation of phagocytosis," *Arzneimittel-Forschung* 41 (1991): 1072–1076.

Wildfeuer, A., and D. Mayerhofer. "The effects of plant preparations on cellular functions in body defense," *Arzneimittel-Forschung* 44 (1994): 361–366.

Chapter 6: The Rest of the Herbal Medicine Chest

Bergner, P. *The Healing Power of Echinacea & Goldenseal*. Rocklin, CA: Prima, 1997.

Braunig, B., et al. "Echinacea purpurea root for strengthening the immune response in flu-like infection," *Zeitschrift Phytotherapie* 13 (1992): 7–13.

Brown, D.J. *Herbal Prescriptions for Better Health*. Rocklin, CA: Prima, 1996.

Castleman, M. *The Healing Herbs: The Ultimate Guide to the Curative Power of Nature's Medicines*. New York, NY: Bantam Books, 1995.

Chang, R. "Functional properties of edible mushrooms," *Nutrition Review* 54 (1996): S91–93.

Degenring, F.H. "Studies on the therapeutic efficacy of Echinaforce®," *Ganzheits Medizin* 2 (1995): 88–94.

Denyer, C.V., et al. "Isolation of antirhinoviral sesquiterpenes from ginger (Zingiber officinale)," *Journal of Natural Products* 57 (1994): 658–662.

Duke, J.A. *The Green Pharmacy*. Emmaus, PA: Rodale, 1997.

Gassinger, C.A., P. Netter, and G. Wunstel. "A controlled clinical trial for testing the efficacy of the homeopathic drug eupatorium perfoliatum D2 in the treatment of common cold," *Arzneimittel-Forschung* 31 (1981): 732–736.

Hahn, F.E., and J. Ciak. "Berberine," *Antibiotics* 3 (1976): 577–588.

Hu, Z., et al. "Mitogenic activity of (-)-epigallocatechin gallate on B-cells and investigation of its structure-function relationship," *International Journal of Immunopharmacology* 14(8) (1992): 1399–1407.

Hughes, B.G., and L.D. Lawson. "Antimicrobial effects of Allium sativum L. (garlic), Allium ampeloprasum L. (elephant garlic), and Allium cepa L. (onion), garlic compounds and commercial garlic supplement products," *Phytotherapy Research* 5 (1991): 154–158.

Iwata, M., et al. "Prophylactic effect of black tea extract as gargle against influenza," *Journal of the Japanese Association of Infectious Diseases* 71(6) (1997): 487–494.

Koch, H.P., and L.D. Lawson. *Garlic: The Science and Therapeutic Application of Allium sativum L. and Related Species*. Baltimore, MD: Williams & Wilkins, 1996.

Kumazawa, Y, et al. "Activation of peritoneal macrophages by berberine-type alkaloids in terms of induction of cytostatic activity," *International Journal of Immunopharmacology* 6 (1984): 587–592.

Lau, B., et al. "Allium sativum (garlic) and cancer prevention," *Nutrition Research* 10 (1990): 937–948.

Leuttig, B., et al. "Macrophage activation by the polysaccharide arabinogalactan isolated from plant cell cultures of *Echinacea purpurea*," *Journal of the National Cancer Institute* 81 (1989): 669–675.

Li, X.Y. "Immunomodulating Chinese herbal medicines," *Mem Inst Oswaldo Cruz* 86 (1991): 159–164.

Lininger, S., et al. *The Natural Pharmacy.* Rocklin, CA: Prima, 1998.

Mascolo, N., et al. "Ethnopharmacologic investigation of ginger (Zingiber officinale)," *Journal of Ethnopharmacology* 27 (1989): 129–140.

Mishra, S., H. Kumar, and D. Sharma. "How do mothers recognize and treat pneumonia at home?", *Indian Pediatrics* 31 (1994): 15–18.

Mitscher, L.A., and V. Dolby. *The Green Tea Book.* Garden City Park, NY: Avery Publishing Group, Inc., 1998.

Mukoyama, A., et al. "Inhibition of rotavirus and enterovirus infections by tea extracts," *Japanese Journal of Medical Science and Biology* 44 (1991): 181–186.

Nakayama, M., et al. "Inhibition of the infectivity of influenza virus by tea polyphenols," *Antiviral Research* 21 (1993): 289–299.

Nakayama, M., et al. "Inhibition of the infectivity of influenza virus by black tea extract," *Journal of the Japanese Association of Infectious Diseases* 68(7) (1994): 824–829.

Okada, K., et al. "Identification of antimicrobial and antioxidant constituents from licorice of Russian and Xinjiang origin," *Chemistry and Pharmacology Bulletin* 37 (1989): 2528–2530.

Okuyama, E., et al. "Usnic acid and diffractaic acid as analgesic and antipyretic components of Usnea diffracta," *Planta Medica* 61 (1995): 113–115.

Roesler, J., et al. "Application of purified polysaccharides from cell cultures of the plant Echinacea purpurea to test subjects mediates activation of the phagocyte system," *International Journal of Immunopharmacology* 13 (1991): 931–941.

Sahelian, R., and D. Gates. *Stevia: Cooking With Nature's No-calorie Sweetener.* Garden City Park, NY: Avery Publishing Group, Inc., 1999.

Scaglione, F., and B. Lund. "Efficacy in the treatment of the common cold of a preparation containing an echinacea extract," *International Journal of Immunotherapy* 11 (1995): 163–166.

Scaglione, F., et al. "Efficacy and safety of the standardised Ginseng extract G115 for potentiating vaccination against influenza syndrome and protection against the common cold," *Drugs Under Experimental and Clinical Research* 22 (1996): 65–72.

Sugiura, H., et al. "Effects of exercise in the growing stage in mice and of Astragalus membranaceus on immune functions," *Japanese Journal of Hygiene* 47 (1993): 1021–1031.

Tyler, V.E. *The Honest Herbal.* Binghamton, NY: Pharmaceutical Products Press, 1993.

Utsunomiya, T., et al. "Glycyrrhizin, an active component of licorice roots, reduced morbidity and mortality of mice infected with lethal doses of influenza virus," *Antimicrobial Agents and Chemotherapy* 41 (1997): 551–556.

Wagner, H., and K. Jurcic. "Immunologic studies of plant combination preparations. In-vitro and in-vivo studies on the stimulation of phagocytosis," *Arzneimittel-Forschung* 41 (1991): 1072–1076.

Weng, X.S. "Treatment of leucopenia with pure Astragalus preparation. An analysis of 115 leucopenic cases," *Chung Kuo Chung Hsi I Chieh Ho Tsa Chih* 15 (1995): 462–464.

Yoshida, Y., et al. "Immunomodulating activity of Chinese medicinal herbs and Oldenlandia diffusa in particular," *International Journal of Immunopharmacology* 19 (1997): 359–370.

Zakay-Rones, Z., et al. "Inhibition of several strains of influenza virus in vitro and reduction of symptoms by an elderberry extract (Sambucus nigra L.) during an outbreak of influenza B

Panama," *Journal of Alternative and Complementary Medicine* 1 (1995): 361–369.

Zhao, K.W., and H.Y. Kong. "Effect of Astragalan on secretion of tumor necrosis factors in human peripheral blood mononuclear cells," *Chung Kuo Chung Hsi I Chieh Ho Tsa Chih* 13 (1993): 263–265.

Chapter 7: Practical Ways to Conquer a Cold and Fight a Flu

Ahmed, F.E. "Toxicological effects of ethanol on human health," *Critical Reviews in Toxicology* 25 (1995): 347–367.

Bendich, A. "Carotenoids and the immune response," *Journal of Nutrition* 119 (1989): 112–115.

Braunig, B. "Echinacea purpurea root for strengthening the immune response in flu-like infection," *Zeitschrift Phytotherapie* 13 (1992): 7–13.

Buffinton, G.D., et al. "Oxidative stress in lungs of mice infected with influenza A virus," *Free Radical Research Communications* 16 (1992): 99–110.

Burton, G.W., et al. "Human plasma and tissue alpha-tocopherol concentrations in response to supplementation with deuterated natural and synthetic vitamin E," *American Journal of Clinical Nutrition* 67 (1998): 669–684.

Chandra, R.K. "Graying of the immune system," *Journal of the American Medical Association* 277 (1997): 1396–1397.

Chandra, R.K. "Effect of vitamin and trace-element supplementation on immune responses and infection in elderly subjects," *Lancet* 340 (1992): 1124–1127.

Cohen, S., et al. "Smoking, alcohol consumption, and susceptibility to the common cold," *American Journal of Public Health* 83 (1993): 1277–1283.

Cohen, S., et al. "Social ties and susceptibility to the common cold," *Journal of the American Medical Association* 277 (1997): 1940–1944.

De Flora, S., L. Carati, and C. Grassi. "Attenuation of influenza-like symptomatology and improvement of cell-mediated immunity with long-term N-acetylcysteine treatment," *European Respiratory Journal* 10 (1997): 1535–1541.

Ferley, J.P., et al. "A controlled evaluation of a homoeopathic preparation in the treatment of influenza-like syndromes," *British Journal of Clinical Pharmacology* 27 (1989): 329–335.

Gassinger, C.A., P. Netter, and G. Wunstel. "A controlled clinical trial for testing the efficacy of the homeopathic drug eupatorium perfoliatum D2 in the treatment of common cold," *Arzneimittel-Forschung* 31 (1981): 732–736.

Glaszious, P.P., et al. "Vitamin A supplementation in infectious diseases: A meta-analysis," *British Medical Journal* 306 (1993): 366–370

Hayek, M.G., et al. "Vitamin E supplementation decreases lung virus titers in mice infected with influenza," *Journal of Infectious Diseases* 17 (1997): 273–276.

Hemilä, H. "Vitamin C supplementation and the common cold. Was Linus Pauling right or wrong?," *International Journal for Vitamin and Nutrition Research* 67 (1997): 329–335.

Hennet, T., E. Peterhans, and R. Stocker. "Alterations in antioxidant defences in lung and liver of mice infected with influenza A virus," *Journal of General Virology* 73 (1992): 39–46.

Hu, Z., et al. "Mitogenic activity of (-)-epigallocatechin gallate on B-cells and investigation of its structure-function relationship," *International Journal of Immunopharmacology* 14(8) (1992): 1399–1407.

Iwata, M., et al. "Prophylactic effect of black tea extract as gargle against influenza," *Journal of the Japanese Association of Infectious Diseases* 71(6) (1997): 487–494.

Kleijnen, J., P. Knipschild, and G. Riet. "Clinical trials of homoeopathy," *British Medical Journal* 302 (1991): 316–323.

Konowalchuk, J., and J.I. Speirs. "Antiviral effect of commerical juices and beverages," *Applied and Environmental Microbiology* 35(6) (1978): 1219–1220.

Kubena, K.S., and D.N. McMurray. "Nutrition and the immune system: A review of nutrient-nutrient interactions," *Journal of the American Dietetic Association* 96 (1996): 1156–1164.

Meydani, S.N., et al. "Vitamin E supplementation and in vivo immune response in healthy elderly subjects," *Journal of the American Medical Association* 277(17) (1997): 1380–1386.

Meydani, S.N., et al. "Antioxidants and immune response in aged persons: overview of present evidence," *American Journal of Clinical Nutrition* 62 (1995): 1462S–1476S.

Mitscher, L.A., and V. Dolby. *The Green Tea Book.* Garden City Park, NY: Avery Publishing Group, Inc., 1998.

Mukoyama, A., et al. "Inhibition of rotavirus and enterovirus infections by tea extracts," *Japanese Journal of Medical Science and Biology* 44 (1991): 181–186.

Nakayama, M., et al. "Inhibition of the infectivity of influenza virus by black tea extract," *Journal of the Japanese Association of Infectious Diseases* 68(7) (1994): 824–829.

Nieman, D.C. "Exercise, upper respiratory tract infection, and the immune system," *Medicine and Science in Sports and Exercise* 26(2) (1994): 128–139.

Pike, J., and R.K. Chandra. "Effect of vitamin and trace element supplementation on immune indices in healthy elderly," *International Journal for Vitamin and Nutrition Research* 65 (1995): 117–120.

Ringsdorf, W.M., et al. "Sucrose, neutrophilic phagocytosis and resistance to disease," *Dental Survey* 52 (1976): 46.

Sahelian, R. *DHEA: A Practical Guide.* Garden City Park, NY: Avery Publishing Group, Inc., 1996.

Santos, M.S., et al. "Natural killer cell activity in elderly men is enhanced by beta-carotene supplementation," *American Journal of Clinical Nutrition* 64 (1996): 772–777.

Sapozhnikov, I.V., et al. "Nonspecific methods of prophylaxis of influenza and other acute respiratory diseases with dibasole and ascorbic acid," *Voprosy Virusologii* 4 (1976): 429–431.

Scaglione, F., et al. "Efficacy and safety of the standardised Ginseng extract G115 for potentiating vaccination against influenza syndrome and protection against the common cold," *Drugs Under Experimental and Clinical Research* 22 (1996): 65–72.

Turner, R.B. "Epidemiology, pathogenesis, and treatment of the common cold," *Annals of Allergy, Asthma, and Immunology* 78 (1997): 531–540.

Turner, R.B., and J. Finch. "Selenium and the immune response," *Proceedings of the Nutrition Society* 50 (1991): 275–285.

Turow, V. "Alternative therapy for colds," *Pediatrics* 100 (1997): 274–275.

West, C.E., et al. "Vitamin A and immune function," *Proceedings of the Nutrition Society* 50 (1991): 251–262.

Zakay-Rones, Z., et al. "Inhibition of several strains of influenza virus in vitro and reduction of symptoms by an elderberry extract (Sambucus nigra L.) during an outbreak of influenza B Panama," *Journal of Alternative and Complementary Medicine* 1 (1995): 361–369.

Chapter 8: Natural Remedies for Specific Symptoms

Andaloro, V.J., D.T. Monaghan, and T.H. Rosenquist. "Dextromethorphan and other N-methyl-D-aspartate receptor antagonists are teratogenic in the avian embryo model," *Pediatric Research* 43 (1998): 1–7.

Braunig, B., et al. "Echinacea purpurea root for strengthening the immune response in flu-like infection," *Zeitschrift Phytotherapie* 13 (1992): 7–13.

Degenring, F.H. "Studies on the therapeutic efficacy of Echinaforce®," *Ganzheits Medizin* 2 (1995): 88–94.

Godfrey, J.C., et al. "Zinc gluconate and the common cold: a controlled clinical study," *Journal of International Medical Research* 20 (1992): 234–236.

Graham, N.M., et al. "Adverse effects of aspirin, acetaminophen, and ibuprofen on immune function, viral shedding, and clinical status in rhinovirus-infected volunteers," *Journal of Infectious Diseases* 162 (1990): 1277–1282.

Grontved, A., et al. "Ginger root against seasickness," *Acta Oto-Laryngologica* 105 (1988): 45–49.

Liapina, L.A., and G.A. Koval'chuk. "A comparative study of the action on the hemostatic system of extracts from the flowers and seeds of the meadowsweet (Filipendula ulmaria [L.] Maxim)," *Izv Akad Nauk Ser Biol* 4 (1993): 625–628.

Kudriashov, B.A., et al. "Heparin from the meadowsweet (Filipendula ulmaria) and its properties," *Izv Akad Nauk Ser Biol* 6 (1991): 939–943.

Mossad, S.B., et al. "Zinc gluconate lozenges for treating the common cold," *Annals of Internal Medicine* 125 (1996): 81–88.

Novick, S.G., et al. "Zinc induced suppression of inflammation in the respiratory tract, caused by infection with human rhinovirus and other irritants," *Medical Hypotheses* 49 (1997): 347–357.

Okuyama, E., et al. "Usnic acid and diffractaic acid as analgesic and antipyretic components of Usnea diffracta," *Planta Medica* 61 (1995): 113–115.

Saketkhoo, K., A. Januszkiewicz, and M.A. Sackner. "Effects of drinking hot water, cold water, and chicken soup on nasal mucus velocity and nasal airflow resistance," *Chest* 74 (1978): 408–410.

Scaglione, F., and B. Lund. "Efficacy in the treatment of the common cold of a preparation containing an echinacea extract," *International Journal of Immunotherapy* 11 (1995): 163–166.

Zakay-Rones, Z., et al. "Inhibition of several strains of influenza virus in vitro and reduction of symptoms by an elderberry extract (Sambucus nigra L.) during an outbreak of influenza B Panama," *Journal of Alternative and Complementary Medicine* 1 (1995): 361–369.

Zeina, B., S. al-Assad, and O. Othman. "Effect of honey versus thyme on Rubella virus survival in vitro," *Journal of Alternative Complementary Medicine* 2 (1996): 345–348.

Index

More than 900,000 copies in print!

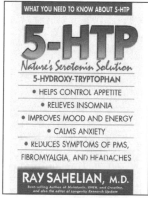

WHAT YOU NEED TO KNOW ABOUT 5-HTP
5-HTP
Nature's Serotonin Solution
5-HYDROXY-TRYPTOPHAN
- HELPS CONTROL APPETITE
- RELIEVES INSOMNIA
- IMPROVES MOOD AND ENERGY
- CALMS ANXIETY
- REDUCES SYMPTOMS OF PMS, FIBROMYALGIA, AND HEADACHES

RAY SAHELIAN, M.D.

224 pp $10.95 Retail

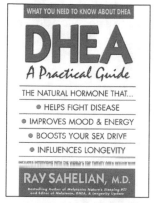

WHAT YOU NEED TO KNOW ABOUT DHEA
DHEA
A Practical Guide
THE NATURAL HORMONE THAT...
- HELPS FIGHT DISEASE
- IMPROVES MOOD & ENERGY
- BOOSTS YOUR SEX DRIVE
- INFLUENCES LONGEVITY

RAY SAHELIAN, M.D.

176 pp $9.95 Retail

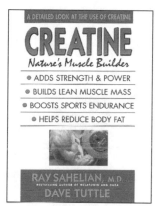

A DETAILED LOOK AT THE USE OF CREATINE
CREATINE
Nature's Muscle Builder
- ADDS STRENGTH & POWER
- BUILDS LEAN MUSCLE MASS
- BOOSTS SPORTS ENDURANCE
- HELPS REDUCE BODY FAT

RAY SAHELIAN, M.D.
DAVE TUTTLE

144 pp $10.95 Retail

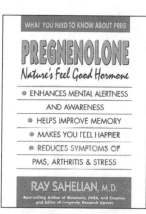

WHAT YOU NEED TO KNOW ABOUT PREG
PREGNENOLONE
Nature's Feel Good Hormone
- ENHANCES MENTAL ALERTNESS AND AWARENESS
- HELPS IMPROVE MEMORY
- MAKES YOU FEEL HAPPIER
- REDUCES SYMPTOMS OF PMS, ARTHRITIS & STRESS

RAY SAHELIAN, M.D.

168 pp $9.95 Retail

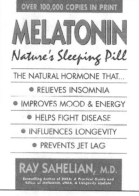

OVER 100,000 COPIES IN PRINT
MELATONIN
Nature's Sleeping Pill
THE NATURAL HORMONE THAT...
- RELIEVES INSOMNIA
- IMPROVES MOOD & ENERGY
- HELPS FIGHT DISEASE
- INFLUENCES LONGEVITY
- PREVENTS JET LAG

RAY SAHELIAN, M.D.

160 pp $9.95 Retail

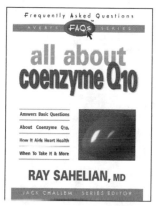

Frequently Asked Questions
AVERY'S FAQs SERIES
all about coenzyme Q10
Answers Basic Questions About Coenzyme Q10.
How It Aids Heart Health
When To Take It & More

RAY SAHELIAN, MD
JACK CHALLEM SERIES EDITOR

96 pp $2.99 Retail

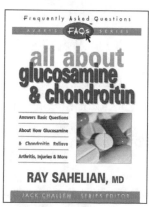

Frequently Asked Questions
AVERY'S FAQs SERIES
all about glucosamine & chondroitin
Answers Basic Questions About How Glucosamine & Chondroitin Relieve Arthritis, Injuries & More

RAY SAHELIAN, MD
JACK CHALLEM SERIES EDITOR

96 pp $2.99 Retail

See website http:\\www.raysahelian.com for latest updates.

To order by credit card call **310–821–2409** (best times are 9:00 a.m. to 5:00 p.m. Pacific time, Monday through Friday) or copy/tear this page and mail in your order. Or by credit card through e-mail: **longrc@aol.com**

Name:_____

Address:_____

City/State/Zip:_____

Telephone:_____

____ copies *5-HTP: Nature's Serotonin Solution*	$10.95	_____
____ copies *Creatine: Nature's Muscle Builder*	$9.95	_____
____ copies *DHEA: A Practical Guide*	$9.95	_____
____ copies *Melatonin: Nature's Sleeping Pill*	$9.95	_____
____ copies *Pregnenolone: Nature's Feel Good Hormone*	$9.95	_____
____ copies *All About Glucosamine & Chondroitin*	$2.99	_____
____ copies *Kava: The Miracle Anti-Anxiety Herb*	$5.99	_____
____ copies *All About Coenzyme Q$_{10}$*	$2.99	_____
____ copies *Lipoic Acid: The Unique Antioxidant*	$3.95	_____
____ copies *Saw Palmetto: Nature's Prostate Healer*	$5.99	_____

Books on stevia and mind-sharpeners coming soon. Call for details.

No shipping charge for the books if mailed to US or Canada.
Shipping (airmail) for overseas: add $6.00 for first book,
and $3.00 for each additional book.   _____

Tax on books shipped to California addresses is 8%.   _____

                                                    Total $_____

Books are shipped promptly.

Please send a check for the total amount to:
          Natural Solutions
          PO Box 12619
          Marina Del Rey, CA 90295

Credit Card #_____   Expires _____

We accept Visa, MC, AE, Diner's Club, Carte Blanche, and JCB cards.

Healthy Habits

are easy to come by—

IF YOU KNOW WHERE TO LOOK!

Get the latest information on:

- **better health • diet & weight loss**
- **the latest nutritional supplements**
- **herbal healing • homeopathy and more**

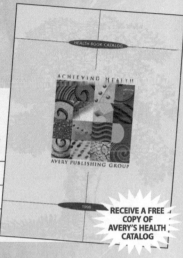

RECEIVE A FREE COPY OF AVERY'S HEALTH CATALOG

COMPLETE AND RETURN THIS CARD RIGHT AWAY!

Where did you purchase this book?

❑ bookstore ❑ health food store ❑ pharmacy
❑ supermarket ❑ other (please specify)_____

Name_____

Street Address_____

City_____State_____Zip_____

GIVE ONE TO A FRIEND ...

Healthy Habits

are easy to come by—

IF YOU KNOW WHERE TO LOOK!

Get the latest information on:

- **better health • diet & weight loss**
- **the latest nutritional supplements**
- **herbal healing • homeopathy and more**

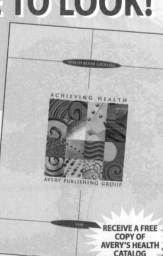

RECEIVE A FREE COPY OF AVERY'S HEALTH CATALOG

COMPLETE AND RETURN THIS CARD RIGHT AWAY!

Where did you purchase this book?

❑ bookstore ❑ health food store ❑ pharmacy
❑ supermarket ❑ other (please specify)_____

Name_____

Street Address_____

City_____State_____Zip_____

Avery Publishing Group
120 Old Broadway
Garden City Park, NY 11040

Avery Publishing Group
120 Old Broadway
Garden City Park, NY 11040